Daniel L. Davis

Your Angry Child
A Guide for Parents

Your Angry Child
A Guide for Parents

THE HAWORTH PRESS
Titles of Related Interest

How Institutions Are Shaping the Future of Our Children: For Better or for Worse? edited by Catherine N. Dulmus and Karen M. Sowers

Emotions and the Family edited by Richard A. Fabes

Community Interventions to Create Change in Children edited by Lorna H. London

Psychoanalytic Approaches to the Treatment of Children and Adolescents: Tradition and Transformation edited by Jerrold R. Brandell

Child Mental Health: Exploring Systems of Care in the New Millennium edited by David A. Dosser Jr., Dorothea Hadron, Susan McCammon, and John Y. Powell

Unbroken Homes: Single-Parent Mothers Tell Their Stories by Wendy Anne Paterson

Innovative Mental Health Interventions for Children: Programs That Work edited by Steven I. Pfeiffer and Linda A. Reddy

The Aggressive Adolescent: Clinical and Forensic Issues by Daniel L. Davis

Diverse Families, Competent Families: Innovations in Research and Preventive Intervention Practice edited by Janet F. Gillespie and Judy Primavera

The Effect of Children on Parents, Second Edition by Anne-Marie Ambert

Teenage Runaways: Broken Hearts and "Bad Attitudes" by Laurie Schaffner

Parents, Children, and Adolescents: Interactive Relationships and Development in Context by Anne-Marie Ambert

Making Families Work and What To Do When They Don't: Thirty Guides for Imperfect Parents of Imperfect Children by Bill Borcherdt

Emerging School-Based Approaches for Children with Emotional and Behavioral Problems: Research and Practice in Service Integration edited by Robert J. Illback and Michael Nelson

Your Angry Child
A Guide for Parents

Daniel L. Davis

The Haworth Press®
New York • London • Oxford

Published by

© 2004 by The Haworth Press, Inc. All rights reserved. No part of this work may be reproduced or utilized in any form or by any means, electronic or mechanical, including photocopying, microfilm, and recording, or by any information storage and retrieval system, without permission in writing from the publisher. Printed in the United States of America.

The Haworth Press, Inc., 10 Alice Street, Binghamton, NY 13904-1580.

AUTHOR'S NOTE
The clinical examples and case histories presented in this book are derived from actual case histories. However, all possible identifying information has been masked and modifications have been made to ensure the anonymity of the individuals portrayed. Although the resulting case histories accurately illustrate and reflect the type of case discussed, any similarity to an actual person, as a result of the changes made, is purely coincidental.

Cover design by Jennifer M. Gaska.

Library of Congress Cataloging-in-Publication Data

Davis, Daniel Leifeld.
    Your angry child : a guide for parents / Daniel L. Davis.
        p. cm.
    Includes bibliographical references and index.
    ISBN 0-7890-1223-5 (hard : alk. paper)—ISBN 0-7890-1224-3 (soft : alk. paper)
    1. Anger in children. 2. Anger in adolescence. 3. Parent and child. 4. Child psychology. 5. Adolescent psychology. I. Title.

BF723.A4D38 2004
649' .153—dc21

                                                                                2003009815

For Lucinda

You are the rose of my winter,

a dance of beauty

in a white cold world

A touch of color

in a time of darkness

that wraps and falls around

the lonely sky

Finding there within

a tapestry of spring

ABOUT THE AUTHOR

Daniel L. Davis, PhD, is a psychologist with Tennenbaum and Associates in Columbus, Ohio, providing forensic consultation and mental health services for children, adolescents, and adults. In addition, Dr. Davis has been a consulting psychologist with Netcare Forensic Psychiatry Services and has consulted with the Columbus Children's Hospital's Behavioral Health Department. Dr. Davis has authored three books and has authored or co-authored numerous professional articles and manuscripts. He appears regularly in local media.

Dr. Davis has served as Clinical Director for Mental Health Services in the Central Ohio Cluster of the Ohio Department of Rehabilitation and Correction. Prior to this position, he was Clinical Director of the Buckeye Ranch, a comprehensive residential and community-based youth treatment center in Columbus. He has also served as Supervising Psychologist in the Timothy B. Moritz Forensic Unit, a maximum-security inpatient forensic psychiatric hospital. Dr. Davis has also held consulting positions with the Ohio Department of Mental Health, the Ohio Department of Youth Services, and the Kentucky Cabinet for Human Services. As a junior in college, he founded and served as the first Director of Concord Counseling Services, a comprehensive mental health center in Westerville, Ohio.

Dr. Davis is a Fellow of the American College of Forensic Psychology and holds an academic appointment in the Department of Psychiatry of the Ohio State University. He is a co-founder of the National Forum on Residential Treatment of Sexually Traumatized Youth. He has testified in over 2,500 juvenile, criminal, and civil cases and he lectures and consults both nationally and internationally.

CONTENTS

Preface

As I reviewed this manuscript, I realized that it is one result of more than thirty years of working with children and families and the study of how to do that. I was struck by how quickly the years have passed. Some of those years were part-time enterprises, some full-time. What struck me was not so much the time but that thirty years ago I sat with a group of fellow college students in a telephone counseling center, taking calls from frantic parents about their teenagers and from angry teens who firmly believed that their parents were the enemy, just like any other adult. Parents liked the counseling center because the counselors were just a little older than the kids. Kids liked us because we were just a little older than them. We could connect.

Now, I am a lot older than both, as my twenty-four-year-old son likes to remind me when he returns home from his graduate studies in psychology. Some of what we thought we knew all those years ago has held up. Much, thankfully, has been discarded. Much more has been learned in the scientific and clinical study of anger. I hope in this work to take that which has been learned in the scientific study of anger and that which I have learned in these years of working with families and kids and combine them into an understandable and helpful book.

No book, especially this one, can be a substitute for an involved, knowing, and caring professional. The purpose of this text is not to replace the involvement of a therapist but to augment. If your child has some or many of the problems discussed here and those problems are interfering with your child's ability to become fully the person he or she can be, or if those problems are causing family difficulties, I urge you to seek help. Often, the first person parents can turn to is their family physician or pediatrician. These doctors are familiar with local resources and can also evaluate for possible physical problems that may either contribute to or worsen the anger problem. If you do not have a physician or need to look elsewhere, look to your local mental health association or college or university. If you have insurance, often your employer's employee assistance program (EAP) or health insurance provider will have a listing of therapists in your area, as will your state psychological association. Many resources are available. The first step, seeking out the help, is the hardest. Help is waiting for the asking.

Acknowledgments

There is a strange paradox in putting forth acknowledgments. Most authors that I know do as I do: write the acknowledgments last. Acknowledgments are the final chapter that is most often placed at the front of the work. This is not the only paradox. These last written words typically honor persons who shaped and influenced us early in our lives, long before we sat down at a keyboard and hoped to find a word or two of value. The reason that we acknowledge, I think, is that those words of value come not so much from us but from what we have learned from others. I am not certain of other writers, but as for me, I am sure. Words of acknowledgment are but a poorly painted portrait of what these people gave to me in the course of my life. But words of acknowledgment are all that are available to me now, and I shall use them.

Simply put, this book could not have been written had I not had the honor of studying under Dr. Henry Leland. Dr. Leland taught me that above all else, we should seek out the health of our clients. I recall vividly the day he told us that any first-year graduate student could diagnose psychopathology, but it took a clinician to find strengths. I try always to remember that. Thank you, Henry.

The other acknowledgment in this book is to my family, my parents, my brother Tom, my sister Judy, my Aunt Nannie, and my Uncle John, all of whom give me strength and the certain knowledge (that I have learned from direct experience) that when all else goes away, my family will not. There are those in my family who are no longer here in the physical sense, my beloved Aunt Bebelle and my grandparents. I learned from them in ways that cannot help but be seen in this writing. Whatever good this work does for someone—and I hope that it will—no amount of science, training, and clinical development could ever replace the life lessons taught to me so lovingly by those to whom I am blood. I thank them. I wish to extend my sincere thanks and admiration to my editor, Dawn Krisko, Senior Production Editor of The Haworth Press for her innumerable improvements to this manuscript. Thank you, Dawn.

Last, there are two who have kept me going. One is my dear Lucinda, who knows already the words I would write. I am certain she prefers to hear rather than read them, so I will leave it at that. The second is my son Josh. Josh, no matter what, I am and always will be so very proud to be your father.

Introduction

When counselors work with children, teenagers, and their families, it is not unusual to encounter some resistance from the youth at first. This is especially the case with kids who feel that the problem isn't with them but really is because their parents are (choose one or all): (1) too strict, (2) too weird, (3) different from all the other parents in the school, (4) totally nonunderstanding, or (5) from some other century or planet. Karl was a youth such as this. A little matter about getting suspended from middle school for the fourth time due to fighting had resulted in what seemed to him to be a totally torturous and unnecessary trip to my office. Not unlike many kids with conduct problems, Karl was not the most verbal—in fact, he was mostly silent, except in certain confrontational family situations when he made up for all of his previous "dead air" in no time at all.

Karl was all about creating dead air in my office. And that's what he did: silently sat there, not responding to anything I had to say. This was not all that unique. But Karl, eager to prove his mastery of the art of being oppositional and defiant, carried it one better. He sat with his back to me throughout the first two sessions. During the first session, when I attempted to interview "Karl's back," there was no response. During the next session, when I continued my discussion by beginning, "Good afternoon, Karl's Back. How are you doing today?" I heard a muffled snicker or two. Later that session, when I invited Karl's Back to sit in on a meeting with his parents while I talked about Karl, he was unable to resist and "gave his back the boot" and participated in a rather animated fashion in the meeting. From then on, save a few times when he would come into my office, flop on my couch, and cover his head with a throw pillow, we got along rather well.

I learned that he had been diagnosed as ADHD (attention-deficit hyperactivity disorder) in the second grade. Karl had been on a variety of medications, refused them all, and was no longer taking anything. He was quite bright and tended to get bored very easily. This boredom would result in his getting into some kind of trouble at school. The school would report this to his exasperated parents, who would drag Karl first to the pediatrician's office for new medication, then to one counselor or another, and, finally, to the police. All of this was in a vain hope to "just get him to listen." The problem was, he did listen. He just didn't agree with what he heard. He also had some tried-and-true ways to successfully demonstrate his displeasure.

It took awhile, but I worked with the parents and helped them to regain control, choose their battles to fight, as well as to not be afraid to be authorities and to set limits and boundaries. I also worked hard with Karl, building on his strengths of a fascinating combination of athletic abilities and artistic sensitivities and talent. He tested my limits and found that the limits were,

1

this time, real. He began to see that arguing and being defiant not only didn't work but also cost him. Karl was able to discover within himself that he was good at something, that he could succeed. Once he learned that, he did succeed.

This is not to say that Karl is now without problems. I wish there were miracle cures, but there really aren't. Karl is much less angry; he really is now "just your basic teenager." Really, that's a good thing. Karl is, after all, a pretty good kid. He and his family still have their moments, but they love each other and they work things through. And that's a pretty good thing too.

That's what this book is about: helping parents and kids who are angry with one another and who can't seem to get along no matter what. It's for parents of kids who seem to always be in some sort of trouble. It's for parents who are worried that their kids are on that path. No miracles can be found here—just some basic, hopefully understandable ideas. Probably some of what you will read, you will remark to yourself, "I knew that." When I used to teach child psychology at a local college, I would tell my students, only half jokingly, that "Developmental (child and adolescent) psychology is really only the scientific study and application of what your grandmother told you." But with all due respect to our collective grandmothers, we have learned a few new things along the way. So, with their permission, let us build upon what they told us. Chapters 2 and 3 introduce, or reacquaint you with, concepts of child development and the development of anger. After that, the chapters become more practical and specific in focus.

Chapter 1

The Impact of Anger

AGGRESSION AND HOSTILITY IN TODAY'S SOCIETY

From what is heard on radio and seen on television or even in a casual look at the newspapers, it seems that hostility and aggression are perhaps the most common forms of interaction between people in today's society. We encounter stories of assault, random aggression, and other attacks on persons daily. It appears as if we live in a world that is increasingly terrifying and out of control. Through the media, we learn of youth that, after patterns of previously unseen "cues" or "warnings," commit some horrifically violent act. Other youth, for no apparent reason, seemingly erupt and seriously injure or kill someone. Even many mental health and social service professionals publicly report that these violent, antisocial youth are beyond any help and can only be removed from the community. We see their images, hear their names, and shudder at what has happened.

We fear that our own children might become victims of a violent act. Or, even more frightening, we fear that they may act in some violent manner and hurt others. We look across our dining room table and there sits an angry, defiant preteenager or teenager and we worry about what is or could be happening. We remember when we could hold them in just one arm, and remember how they used to love to ride atop our shoulders. We recall all those things and wonder, *How did it get to this point?* Or more urgently, *What can we do?* According to the U.S. Department of Justice (Snyder and Sickmund, 1999), one out of every 290 youth between the ages of ten and seventeen was arrested for a violent crime. Although there may be periodic drops, youth aggression remains at a historically high and unacceptable level in our communities. In response, many locales and states have

3

become far more restrictive when dealing with these youth. Aggressive and antisocial youth are now sent to juvenile correctional facilities at an earlier age and often for much longer periods of time. A substantial number of youth are now serving time in adult correctional facilities. Further, many states have lowered the age at which a juvenile may be transferred to the jurisdiction of the adult courts and subsequently sent to an adult correctional facility. According to the U.S. Department of Justice, in 2000 there were nearly 10,000 juveniles in adult prisons or jails. According to trends in correctional populations, there may eventually be more youth incarcerated in adult facilities than in juvenile correctional institutions.

Although crime statistics suggest a recent drop in the number of violent crimes reported, this is a misleading statistic. Many youthful perpetrators of violent crimes who are now either incarcerated in adult or juvenile correctional facilities will someday be discharged. Without proper interventions throughout incarceration, when they do leave they may be as violent and most likely more so than when they entered the system.

THE EFFECT OF AGGRESSION AND HOSTILITY ON THE FAMILY

As frightening as the crime statistics are, for most of us they remain in the abstract. What matters most, of course, is what happens in our cities, in our neighborhoods, and in our families. In our homes, we are no longer insulated from the effect of hostility and aggression. Family life can become almost engulfed by an angry and difficult child. Much is said about the effect of the family upon the youth, but it works both ways. The angry and difficult child can have a substantial and negative impact upon the rest of the family. Then, in response, members of the family rejoin back in an angry way and the youth becomes even more angry and oppositional. The cycle repeats over and over until one side (generally the parent) becomes exhausted and gives in.

In other situations, circumstances may become explosive to the extent that others outside of the family must intervene. This cycle will repeat until something stops it. That something can be positive or negative. If positive, such as learning how to solve problems without fighting, the family can regroup and learn from what happened in a manner to prevent or lessen the possibility of the problem happening again. If the intervention is negative, such as an arrest, then matters can become even worse. When those negative consequences do happen, families look for something or someone to blame. Often, parents blame themselves. The mental health field has had a long history of looking for causes or blames that masquerade as exploitations. This is changing, but it is probably not soon or well-known enough to allow us to build upon what is right rather than blame what is wrong in families.

There was a time when a person's unconscious mind was blamed for his or her negative actions. It was thought that much of what a person did was the result of his or her unconscious reactions to what happened in early childhood. He or she wasn't responsible for what he or she did. After all, the true cause of behavior happened years ago. How could the person be held accountable for actions that really resulted from the actions, years ago, of his or her parents?

Thankfully, the mental health field doesn't think that way anymore. Clinicians know that people are responsible for their choices and their actions, including the youth.

There was another time, maybe even darker, when the problems of society were blamed upon "bad seeds," or genetically inferior humans. Not only did this lead to horrific examples of genocide in Europe and sterilization of minorities in the United States, it also formed (and probably still contributes to) prejudice and discrimination. Although no rational behavioral scientist disagrees today that genetics play an important role (e.g., studies of the behaviors of twins reared miles apart who act in almost identical fashion), we recognize that it is the interaction between a person's genes and his or her environment that determines how that person will act. This "interactive" model has been the standard, but a rise in genetic research raises again the possibility that valuable scientific findings will be misunderstood or deliberately misinterpreted by those who wish to justify and further their own prejudices.

Why are kids so angry and why do some become violent? There is no single answer to such a complex question. Anger is an emotion that can have very positive or negative consequences. Often, the nature of the consequence depends upon how anger is expressed. For example, positive anger can lead to social change. In the middle of the twentieth century, African Americans used their anger, a result of years of oppression, to dramatically change society. We have all benefited from that change. Without that anger, we would have lost much in our society. At an individual level, a person can be angry at a situation or circumstance and with constructive expression of that anger make a meaningful change. Films such as *Norma Rae* (1979) or *Erin Brockovich* (2000) tell the heroic struggles of individuals who used their anger to make changes in their lives and in the lives of others. At a not so dramatic level, we can learn to channel and redirect our anger into all sorts of positive efforts. Sports, for example, can be a means by which a young person can funnel his or her aggression and anger and learn habits of self-control and self-confidence.

RESISTANCE AND OPPOSITIONAL BEHAVIOR

Responses to anger are not always direct. Indirect expressions can also be both positive and negative. Anger can be internalized and result in a number of health problems such as heart disease, high blood pressure, and depression. Anger can show itself in negativism and defiance. It can also be indirectly expressed in a positive way. Take for example the writings of Henry David Thoreau, whose treatise on civil disobedience led to the nonviolent revolutions of Mohandas K. Gandhi and Martin Luther King Jr. In these circumstances, anger at injustice and oppression resulted in active but nonviolent resistance that eventually overcame the forces of repression and injustice in society.

All of this philosophy does little good when your child throws a major temper tantrum at the grocery store. Rather than dwell on the meaning of your child's screams, you really just want the tantrum to stop. Later on, you can see if that particular explosion over the lack of a favorite item at that store has much to do with the ultimate meaning of life. But for now you think, *Could we please just get this kid to calm down?*

Chapter 2

The Workings of Anger

TEMPERAMENT AND ANGER

Lucifer

Karen and Jim had the perfect child. Karen's pregnancy and the delivery went smoothly. Little Betsy wasn't really perfect, but she was so good that it seemed as if she had slept through the night very quickly and always woke with a warm and loving smile. Why, little Betsy was such an ideal infant that she not only was asked to pose for all sorts of infant modeling jobs, she toilet trained herself while helping the photographer set the camera angles. Or so it seemed. Parenthood was such a joy to Karen and Jim that they just couldn't stop at one baby. Since, after all, they had the perfect baby, why not have another? When one child is this good, two can only be better. (Experienced parents of more than one child, please hold your comments until the end of this introduction.)

So, Karen and Jim produced another child, certain that any other baby was destined to live forever in the shadows of their progeny. Just as before, Karen sailed through her pregnancy. The delivery went so easily that Karen later remarked that she could have fit it in between her aerobic lessons and mowing the yard. It was only later that the horrible truth fell upon them: theirs was not the pretender to the throne of the perfect child. Not even close. Instead, it was clear that they had brought into their family the "Infant from Hades." Never was there a fussier child. Never was there a child who could instinctively know as well the very moment either one of the parents had fallen asleep and would then let loose with a demonic cry that not only shook the parents from their beds but the neighbors as well. This child never slept at regular times. Night would become evening, and just when Karen and Jim adjusted to that, young Lucifer would decide to become an early riser. Not only did Lucifer not breast-feed, his approach to formula was more like a grumpy gourmet who never found a meal worth eating. But no gourmet was as adept at projectile vomiting as young Lucifer, who rivaled Davy Crockett in aim and accuracy. And these were his good days!

In between nearly hourly diaper changes, constant crying, and dodging of partially digested food, Karen and Jim wondered how they could have so very different children. Weren't their genes the same as before? Didn't they act the same way toward lovely little Betsy as they did toward young Lucifer? "How could these two children be so very different?" they wondered aloud while driving to the doctor's office for Jim's vasectomy.

The story of poor Jim and Karen most likely resonates with many people. Parents often struggle with trying to understand how it is that one child born to the same family can be so very different from a sibling. Certain differences can be understood, but it can be quite puzzling when the differences are great. Parents often blame themselves (or accept the blame of others) for the difficult child. They are given remedy after remedy for the uncooperative infant. They dive into self-help books and pray that some television talk show has a child-development expert who can answer the question once and for all, someone who can simply tell them what to do.

What did they do to deserve this fate? Often, the answer is nothing. Children are not born the same. Nor, as once believed, are they born as "blank slates" ready to be molded and shaped by the behaviors of their parents. Now we understand that children come "prewired emotionally" into this world. Some are born with an easy, agreeable temperament, and others are just the opposite. They are difficult, challenging, and sometimes exhausting. This is not to say that the actions of the parents have nothing to do with the temperament of a child—far from it. In fact, the emotions of the child affect the parents, who then respond back to the child, who then responds to the response, and so forth. One clearly influences the other. There is no real way to ever truly separate fully the influences of nature and nurture.

However, there really are differences in children in their basic emotional state or temperament. *Temperament* is defined as the inborn ways or repertoire of traits with which a child is equipped to deal with his or her environment. Although we are born with these basic traits and there is some continuity throughout life, temperament can be modified throughout the child's development. This is especially the case with interactions, or the lack of them, with the primary caregiver early in the child's life.

Child-development research provides three basic categories of temperament (understanding of course that no one child is a "clean fit" in just one category): easy, difficult, and slow to warm up. Differences between these types are clearly distinguishable from birth. The easy child is generally happy, flexible, and regular in his or her behavior. He or she gets along well with nearly everyone and presents few problems to parents and, later on, to other adults (e.g., teachers). The difficult child is starkly the opposite. As an infant and later on as a young child and adolescent, he or she can be intense, demanding, inflexible, and very moody. The third group, slow to warm up, does not respond very well to changes in environment, but his or her reactions are not intense. The child generally has a low activity level and tends to withdraw from new situations and people.

Does that mean that once children are born, that's it? Nothing can change? No, of course not. Parents can and should work with their children's temperament. Although it will most likely be the case that parents can't make major changes, a lot can be done. This knowledge is so very important because children who are chronically oppositional and defiant often have problems regulating or managing their moods. They can be taught to *manage* how they feel, even if they can't *change* how they feel. For example, children can be taught to express their frustration in ways that aren't so destructive. This can and ideally does begin early. If children are "difficult," parents need to work hard at being consistent in discipline. Although it can be hard at times, when it is time to discipline, parents should try to be objective and nonemotional with difficult children. As we will see later in this book, an excellent skill for parents of oppositional children to learn is to not get caught in power-and-control struggles. Conversely, with slow-to-warm-up children, parents need to remember to allow them to move at their own pace; gentle encouragement is best.

Sometimes, parents and teachers can change the environment of the children to make it so that they do the best they can. Children who are difficult in temperament also have a very difficult time coping with environments that change frequently and are unstructured. Thus, parents of difficult children would want to educate teachers to make sure that classrooms are structured in a manner that is consistent and fair. This is not to say that easy children are without problems. Sometimes easy children feel the need to please others and to reduce conflict. As adults, we know that this is not always possible. But children, with their limited range of experience and tendency to internalize, will often blame themselves when they fail to solve conflict between two difficult peers.

Understanding temperament is important for parents because it forms the developmental basis for our emotions. One of the most basic and perhaps essential emotions of human beings is anger. We all know what anger is. We have felt when we're angry, and when others are angry with us. Anger is a basic and necessary human emotion that is completely healthy and usually normal. It is not so much the anger that causes problems. It is, rather, what we do when angry that can result in difficulties. When anger is expressed in a healthy way, it can lead to positive change and psychological growth. Sometimes, it can just be a fleeting annoyance in our lives. Other times, it can be a destructive rage. It is when anger becomes constant or gets out of control that relationships and quality of life suffer.

Children are not born knowing how to handle their anger. They learn through trial and error, through teaching, and, most important, by observing others. Many parents are proud to see their children act the same way that they do. However, when they haven't learned to handle their anger, parents wish their children could do better than they did.

THINKING AND ANGER

Children are born with different temperaments, and they respond differently to situations. Some children simply become angry much easier than others. The child with the difficult temperament is the child who most likely has a shorter fuse. The child who is slow to warm up will be just as likely to be slow to anger. In much the same fashion, the easy child may not perceive the circumstance or situation in a way likely to cause anger.

In each case, what seems to be most important is not so much whether the child becomes angry but what the child does with that anger. Anger and aggression are not the same thing. Anger is a feeling, and aggression is a behavior. Sometimes children act in an aggressive way because they are angry. In fact, aggression may be the very first way that they learn how to respond to their anger. Aggression is an instinctive and natural way to respond. But of course that doesn't mean aggression is the only way to respond. There are many other ways, some healthy, some not.

It is even possible for some individuals to act in a very aggressive way and not feel the least bit of anger. A good illustration of nonemotional aggression would be the athlete who channels aggression into superior performance. Because of this believed link between aggression and anger, parents can confuse them and teach their children to not respond at all to perfectly justifiable feelings of anger. If children are not taught a variety of ways of responding then they have a very limited repertoire of available behaviors. In a sense, it is like the old Russian proverb, "To a hammer the whole world is a nail."

What can we change about temperament? We know that it is not so much how we feel about things but how we think about them that determines how we respond. For example, one person may bump into another person. The person who is bumped can interpret that bump in one of two ways. If the person feels the bump was an accident, perhaps the feeling of mild annoyance at most will result. If the person feels the bump was on purpose, then an entirely different emotion may result. We know that some people habitually look at a situation in a manner more likely to result in anger. Simply put, some of us walk around with chips on our shoulders all the time. Why are we like that? There are lots of reasons, but most of the time it is because life experiences have taught us to look at the world in that manner. The following text explores how this happens by looking first at the development of thinking (or cognition), and then the development of angry thought styles in children.

THE DEVELOPMENT OF THOUGHT PROCESSES

Jean Piaget formulated a model of cognitive growth that has become a landmark in child psychology. Piaget observed the development of his two nieces as they learned about their world and stated that human cognitive development builds from the simple to the complex. Development involves a continuous process of change and adaptation in the manner in which we deal with our environment. Development is the result of four factors: maturation, experience, social transmission, and the process of equilibrium. *Maturation* is the unfolding of the genetic blueprints in our life: some things develop following a natural plan that rests in our genes. For example, as a child grows older, he or she develops secondary sexual characteristics when puberty occurs. These physical changes follow a prescribed genetic plan. They happen without our doing anything consciously. But, of course, there is more to adolescence than simply physical change. We grow and experience new situations.

Experience refers to the active process of interaction between the child and the environment. As the youth grows, he or she participates in many new experiences. To illustrate, not only does puberty cause physical change, but as teens physically mature, they also are exposed to many new situations. They become interested in the world outside of their homes. Peers become more important influences, often even more than family members. This interaction with other new people can cause a change in the personality of the teen. Then, the new aspect of that personality is tested on the outside world. The behaviors of the youth affect others around him or her. The reactions of those affected influence whether or how that new aspect of personality will influence later behaviors of the teen. Take for example cigarette smoking. The teen may try this behavior and meet with approval of his or her peers, finding that it makes him or her seem older, more "cool." In that way, the response of those around the teen causes him or her to want to continue smoking. In contrast, another youth takes up smoking and receives a very negative result from his or her friends, who criticize and make fun of the teen for smoking. Most likely, this youth will quickly stop smoking. Thus, not only did the action (smoking) cause a reaction (approval or disapproval by friends), but that reaction resulted in a change in the youth (continuing or quitting smoking).

This illustration also shows how very important the responses of others are to the development of our thinking and our behavior. We learn from one another. This process is called social transmission. *Social transmission* describes the information and customs passed along from parents and other persons in the environment to children. One important feature of social transmission is the change of influences as children grow. The first influence is the immediate family. Later, as they grow older and experience more of the world, other social influences evolve. A key one of these, of course, is the influence of the media—television, movies, music, and video games—which we will discuss later. But in addition to these influences, growing children develop friends who influence them. Later on, during adolescence, the influence of peers can become stronger than those of the parents (as many parents of teenagers learn, somehow forgetting that the very same thing happened with them).

Last, the process of *equilibrium* describes the nature of human development. For us, balance in our lives is very important. We always look to maintain stability. This need for balance is a basic biological and psychological process of growth. The growing child seeks to maintain a balance between what he or she knows and what he or she is experiencing. In this process of development, there are discrete, different stages of how our thinking processes grow and change. These stages occur in a specific, unchangeable sequence. Each stage is quite different from the others. They must occur in a specific order. A child cannot move from the first to the last stage without passing through all those that lie in between.

How is all of this important to the development of angry kids? The following is a good example. Two-year-old children are still very egocentric or self-focused in their thinking. They have to be in order to survive. To them, the world must revolve around them because they depend upon others to take care of them. Without the involvement of parents or caregivers, toddlers could not survive on their own. Thus, being egocentric is not being "selfish"; rather, it is vital to growth and survival. But having two egocentric kids in the same play space can be a harrowing experience. Try this little experiment. Take a couple of two-year-olds and give each one his or her favorite plaything. Then, try to make them share. It probably won't happen. If it does, it won't be for long. That doesn't mean the kids are selfish. Rather, they are just being what they should psychologically be at that age. But this can most certainly result in frustration for the caregiver who does not understand how kids of this age think. Kids will learn to share, but not until they are psychologically ready to learn.

As children develop, they create cognitive schemes or methods of dealing with the environment that can be generalized to many situations. To illustrate, an abused child will frequently develop a scheme of the world as a hostile and dangerous place. Thus, each time the child views a new situation, he or she views it as potentially threatening and harmful. As another example, racial prejudice could be partially understood as the application of a fixed schema to all persons who have specific characteristics. Thus, prejudice is to a great extent understood as ignorance and an unwillingness to learn. A person takes fixed (and usually negative) beliefs (schema) about a specific group of people and applies them without regard for the truthfulness or validity of those beliefs.

When a child takes in the environment, he or she must adapt or adjust to the environment in order to survive. Adaptation involves two processes that complement each other: assimilation and accommodation. *Assimilation* takes place when newly learned information is altered to fit existing patterns of thought. For example, the young child may describe all men as "daddy." As another illustration, it may be believed by some that there was once a requirement that all graduate students in the 1970s drive a beat-up Volkswagen Beetle. I was no exception, and my then-two-year-old son knew the vehicle as "Daddy's bug car." Once while driving our other car, we drove past a similar Volkswagen. Josh became hysterical, believing that someone else was driving his father's car.

This process of assimilation is not limited to just children. To continue with the Volkswagen example, these cars had a reputation for being quite easy to repair. For me, a Volkswagen repair should have been easy. My family, on my father's side, had a long history with the railroad. My grandfather was a railroad mechanic who advanced to running the railroad roundhouse. When my father was a teen, my grandfather took him to a junkyard to find a vehicle. They then rebuilt it and my father continues to treasure the memory of his Model A Ford. If development were strictly genetic, it would stand to reason that I, too, would be able to repair mechanical things. But try as I did, the only thing I successfully learned to do was the relatively simple act of tuning up the engine. This worked wonderfully when the problem was the lack of a tune-up. Unfortunately, beyond changing the oil, it was the only thing I could do. So, when the brakes went out, I tuned the engine. Then, as I crashed into the wall because I could not stop the car, I could at least listen to the purring of that well-tuned engine.

Accommodation takes place when a person must modify existing thought patterns to fit new information. It is, in essence, a new way of thinking. Youth who have been chronically abused, to return to this example, typically are unable to easily accommodate new social information. Rather, they will persistently and often illogically, to an outside observer, attempt to assimilate social information into pre-existing structures. Thus, the well-meaning adult who attempts to hug a distraught abused child may be unpleasantly surprised by the child's negative and potentially angry reaction.

Although each stage has age ranges, these stages are approximate and are best seen as guideposts. Further, as a result of trauma or some type of developmental disability or influence, a person may stay fixated within one stage and not progress to the next. This is a central point in the understanding of angry behavior. Over the years, research has demonstrated that angry persons think differently than nonangry persons. Not only do they think differently in terms of content (more angry fantasies, for example), they also think in a qualitatively different way. As will be seen in Chapter 6, the form of their thinking often does not allow for the more abstract concepts that nonangry persons use to stifle or suppress angry impulses.

The stages that I have alluded to throughout this chapter are those of Piaget. Piaget's first stage, *sensorimotor,* takes place between birth and two years of age. The infant explores the world through sight, taste, and motor activity. During this period, the child develops *object permanence,* the understanding that people and objects do not disappear merely because they are out of sight.

The second stage, *preoperational,* lasts from ages two through seven, approximately. Children learn that one thing can symbolically stand for another. (A piece of wood can become a toy airplane, for example.) Children of this age are "magical" in their thinking at times, tending to believe that inanimate objects can come to life. Children at this age are quite egocentric, believing that each person sees the world in the same manner as they view it. Once, for example, when I had the flu, young Josh brought me his Winnie-the-Pooh blanket, reasoning that since it made him feel good, it would have the same effect on me. Egocentricity can result in social difficulties. In a much more serious light, when divorce happens while a child is in this cognitive stage, it is easy to see how the child could blame himself or herself for the destruction of the family.

At approximately six to seven years of age, the child moves to the *concrete operations* stage. Here, he or she becomes gradually less egocentric and develops more sophisticated processes of thought, such as conservation (the recognition that a quart of water in a tall pitcher has the same mass as a quart of water in a stout container). The child's thinking remains highly concrete and full of literal interpretations. It is also known that frontal lobe brain-injured persons think in a highly concrete way. The famous Russian neuropsychologist Goldstein once reported an observation in which a brain-injured patient became highly upset upon hearing a physician remark, upon looking out the window during a stormy morning, that "It was a dark day." To the concrete-thinking patient, this was impossible. If it was dark, then it must be night. If it was day, then it could not be dark.

To illustrate how concrete thinking works, the following is a case example taken from a time when I worked with very severely disturbed children in a residential treatment center.

Leon

Leon was a youth of borderline mentally retarded intellectual functioning. His mother had been an alcoholic and he suffered from fetal alcohol syndrome. In addition, he had suffered severe environmental deprivation and abuse during his early childhood. His mother frequently abandoned him and was grossly neglectful of him. He was removed from his home when he was six years old and placed in emergency foster care. Two days later, he set fire to the foster house. The foster parents were both severely burned and their child was killed by smoke asphyxiation. Leon was placed in a specialized, secure residential treatment center.

He adapted well to the highly structured treatment program and seemed to enjoy the rules and order, which he had never before known. Each child at the program had his or her own footlocker to keep those items allowed in the program. To discourage theft, each locker had a small padlock. Some youth that had demonstrated sufficient responsibility were allowed to keep their own key to the lock, rather than having it stored in the staff office.

One of Leon's proudest moments was the day he was given his footlocker key. Rather than carrying it on a string around his neck, as was the manner of the other youth, he managed to obtain a key clip from a staff member who had taken a particular liking to him. This key clip greatly resembled the kind worn by the staff, and Leon took great pride in his clip. The treatment team interpreted his pride as, potentially, visible evidence that he was beginning to identify in a positive manner with staff.

There was one problem. Technically, it was against the rules of the facility for the youth to have such key clips. For some reason never clearly understood, youth that held keys were required to either wear them around their necks or keep them on a ring in their pockets. Leon's team, however, chose to ignore this rule and make a special exception for Leon since it seemed so important to him.

One day, most of the regular staff was away for training. A new staff member, on probation, saw Leon's key clip and knew that youth were not allowed to have such things. He took the clip and kept Leon's key in the staff office. As would be expected, Leon became extremely upset. He became agitated and combative to the degree that he required physical restraint.

The next day, the team returned and was shocked by what had happened. They called Leon into the team meeting to talk about it. They asked him how he felt. He quickly and angrily replied that he wanted to "get back" at the staff member who had taken his key ring. The team, becoming concerned that Leon would assault the staff member, asked Leon just what he was planning to do. In a statement reflecting clear purpose and conviction, Leon stated that he planned to go find the new staff member and take away the staff member's own keys.

Finally, beginning around age twelve and continuing through adolescence (although many parents of teenagers find this hard to believe), the thinking process matures to its highest level. Children are now able to think in a manner termed by Piaget as *formal operations.* This most mature level of thinking results in the youth being able to deal with abstractions, test hypotheses in a mature manner, and understand complex ethical issues. It is, in some sense, why youth become so concerned with matters of principles and hold to rigid absolutes. They have only begun to be able to see these issues and retain certain concrete qualities to their thinking, especially in early portions of formal operations.

MORAL REASONING

Kohlberg, a developmental psychologist, used Piaget's model in the concept of the development of moral reasoning. Early on in our development, we exhibit *preconventional morality.* All actions are seen in strict either/or terms and justice is swift and sure. To illustrate, when a group of four-year-olds were asked about a young boy who had shoplifted some candy and then, on his way home, was struck by a car, the children were quite certain that the child had suffered a direct consequence to his theft. Because he had stolen, the children reasoned, being struck by a car punished him. The next stage, *conventional morality,* is defined by an emphasis upon rules and order. If a person breaks a rule, then he or she must be punished. Justice is a matter of "an eye for an eye." There can be no room for consideration of individual or mitigating circumstances. (If one is twelve years old, therefore, one should not opt for a jury of one's peers.) Kohlberg, of course, believes that some adults have never moved out of this stage of moral reasoning. The last stage, *universal ethical principle,* allows for greater understanding of truths beyond mere rules of conduct. A person at this stage can understand and appreciate the civil disobedience of a Gandhi or a King, for example.

APPRAISAL AND EXPECTATIONS:
DEVELOPING STYLES OF ANGRY THINKING

The way in which we think about situations is linked to the interactive mechanisms of cognitive appraisal and expectations. These are essentially learned perceptual processes. Appraisals are the characteristic ways in which a person views the environment, and expectations are the person's prediction of the outcome of an anticipated behavior. Habitual appraisals and expectations predispose a person to act in a certain way in response to his or her perception of circumstances and to expect that behavior to be either successful or unsuccessful depending upon previous experiences.

Appraisals are how we look at the world. One illustration is the saying about a half of a glass of water. A pessimist looks at the glass and sees it as half empty. An optimist looks at the glass as half full. Why is that? Mostly because of life experiences that have shaped the way he or she looks at things. A person who has had a great deal of disappointment in his or her life will naturally expect more empty glasses than full ones. A child who has experienced many frustrations, losses, or conflicts in his or her life might well look at a situation in a way more likely to result in an angry response. In more drastic circumstances, the angry and aggressive youth sees himself or herself in a threatening world. Often, past experiences of abuse and pain have taught the youth that. He or she has experienced the world to be consistently hostile and expects it to continue as such, believing it to be foolish to be any other way.

Beyond the process of appraisal—how we look at the world—is an action that we do when we think about our world and situations. That action is the process of expectations, what we think about our own behaviors. With young children, an excellent example is the classic story of *The Little Engine That Could.* If you remember this wonderful story, the little engine chugs up the steep hill saying, "I think I can, I think I can." When the little engine finally reaches the top of the hill, the words (or self-talk) change to, "I knew I could." Of course, this is one of the most valuable lessons that parents try to teach their children: that believing in themselves is crucial to success. Sadly, not all kids learn to believe in themselves. Adults who are harsh and critical of them may break their spirit. Such children develop a negative belief system about themselves and encounter new situations with a belief that they will more likely fail than succeed. It is not at all surprising, then, that such children are often angry and frustrated when faced with new situations and experiences.

Expectations can also work to continue negative and angry behavior. If a child becomes angry and throws a temper tantrum and it works, then the child quickly learns that temper tantrums are a handy means to get his or her own way. If you, as an astute two-year-old, decide that you simply don't want to be in that grocery store any longer, then the answer to your problem is simple. You let the world know exactly how you feel. You yell, cry, fuss, toss, and scream—whatever it takes to sufficiently motivate your parent to leave the grocery store. Then, satisfied, you reward your parent-in-training by once again becoming that happy child we all know and love.

A more serious illustration is that of schoolyard bullies. They have learned to get what they want by pushing people around. The problems come when being a bully doesn't work. Bullies don't develop the kinds of social skills that kids who aren't bullies develop. Kids who are bullies don't know how to compromise; they don't know how to delay gratification; and they don't know how to work cooperatively with other children. They don't know these things not because they can't learn them; rather it is because they have never had to develop such skills. For them, aggression works often enough that they can generally get their way by being a bully. They have the expectation that angry, pushy, and aggressive behavior will generally get them what they want.

ANGER AND ATTACHMENT

Jeremy

I was asked to consult on the case of Jeremy, a fifteen-year-old boy who was serving a twenty-years-to-life sentence in an adult prison for the murder of his foster mother. Now in the prison mental health unit, he was very violent and paranoid. I was asked to provide treatment suggestions for him. In such cases, the first thing to do is to review the records of prior treatment. In Jeremy's case, there were volumes. He was the child of an alcoholic mother and an unknown father. Removed from his mother's custody at the age of three months because of neglect, he was placed in the child welfare system. Between the ages of three months and fourteen years, he was placed in twenty-two separate foster homes and treatment facilities. He was never in one setting for longer than one year. He had seven different caseworkers and at least six different psychological evaluations. Before the offense, he was essentially adrift and alone in the foster care system. The day of the murder, he had just arrived at the foster home. He did not know the name of his new foster mother. But for some reason, still known only to him, he stood behind her and stabbed her over fifty times, causing her death. Arrested, bound over from juvenile court, he was tried as an adult and sentenced to potentially spend the rest of his life in prison. His rage made perfect sense to me.

Another crucial area to explore in the understanding of anger is that of attachment. In the eyes of many developmental and child psychologists, the development of healthy attachments is the basis of positive mental health and social relations in children. This understanding came first in the work of John Bowlby who suggested that the pattern of an infant's early attachment to parents would form the basis of all later social relationships. Human beings live in societies and groups. We bond with one another. We have families, organizations, and businesses—many ways that we relate to and help one another. The human infant cannot survive on his or her own. He or she is dependent upon others.

Needs for survival are not just physical. Many years ago, researcher Rene Spitz (1945) studied children in an orphanage. The facility had been updated to what were at the time the most modern methods of care. During the turn of the nineteenth century, physicians had discovered antiseptics and had made amazing advances in the fight against diseases. As a result, this orphanage had modernized by creating a completely antiseptic environment. Each infant was kept alone in a sterile crib, shielded from other children by white sheets around the crib. The caregivers wore gowns, gloves, and masks. The infants began to die at a horrifying rate. Completely confused, the administrators of the foundling home contacted Dr. Spitz, who took away the antiseptic boundaries, made certain that the infants could see and hear one another, and most important, directed the caregivers to hold, touch, and interact with the babies. The children stopped dying.

We are really no different after infancy. Psychologically, we cannot survive without human interaction. Healthy attachments are pivotal to the development of emotionally healthy children. Some children struggle with attachment. They become anxious, afraid, and unwilling to let their caregivers out of sight. Although a degree of separation anxiety is normal and probably essential to survival, some children never seem to gain the self-confidence to allow them to put some distance between themselves and their caregiver. When children who have healthy attachments are put into experimental rooms that allow them to explore, they first go to their mothers who were placed in the center of the room. However, as they gain confidence, they quickly begin to move about and explore the room. In contrast, children with anxious attachments cling and hold on to their mothers. If the mothers attempt to separate or otherwise prod them into exploring, the children react with genuine distress and refuse to leave. Such children often develop personalities that are characterized by fear, doubts, and anxieties.

ANGER AND THE ANTISOCIAL CHILD

In the experiments previously discussed, a third, far more rare kind of attachment is sometimes seen. This child, the unattached child, has never really bonded to any caregiver or any other child. Put in the experimental situation, the child continues on as he or she has done all along, charging about a new situation, caring not who or what gets in his or her way. When the caregiver approaches the child, rather than going to the caregiver for any type of comfort or reassurance, the child shows anger and annoyance at being interrupted from his or her exploration of the new surroundings.

Children who grow up without real attachments or bonds to others are the most likely to develop substantial emotional problems. Often, such children become violent offenders later in life. Not surprisingly, a primary diagnostic criterion for a psychopath or antisocial personality is the lack of any ability to form meaningful and genuine attachments to others. Instead, these criminals either con and manipulate others or eliminate others who are of no use to them. In essence, attachment is the foundation for healthy emotional, moral, and social development.

Thankfully, the Jeremys of the world are rare. But they do exist. In recent years, we have learned through careful developmental study that certain children appear to not be able to develop true relationships with others. From a very early age, they seem unattached, calculating, and lacking in empathy or understanding of the thoughts and feelings of others. As they grow, they remain at an emotional distance from other children and adults. They often seem to lack the usual range of feelings seen in children. Rather, they tend to be cool, often without anxiousness when caught or confronted, and show remorse only when caught or confronted with their misdeeds. The remorse that they do show is easily seen as shallow and more about being caught than feeling genuinely guilty about what they have done. When in such situations, truth for them is simply a tool. When they can lie to avoid responsibility, they will do so. When caught in a lie, they likely will lie again. The truth is told only when there seems to be no other way out of trouble; they will blame others and try to present themselves as helpless victims of circumstances. When punished, they will not learn from the consequence. Punishment serves only to briefly contain them until the next opportunity to misbehave.

Animal Cruelty and Fire Setting

Some of these children have other behaviors that appear to coalesce with antisocial behavior. They frequently are cruel to animals. They go far beyond simple poor judgment or even rough play with the animal and will mistreat and even torture it. Although not all children who mistreat animals grow up to be antisocial adults and not all antisocial adults mistreat animals, the link between animal cruelty and later violent behavior has been clearly demonstrated in psychological research.

A similar way that lack of attachment can be seen is in fire setting. Fire has a life and power of its own. It holds our attention and we seem to truly enjoy having it around. After all, why do many of our houses have fireplaces when we have no need for them to heat our houses? However, for youth who have real significant problems with attachment and often no regard for others, fire can be an effective tool to control and dominate. Fire, once started, cannot be ignored. Children who feel that they have no power over what happens in their lives or who seek revenge quickly learn that adults must respond to a fire.

Donnie

Donnie was a hapless child. He was born to parents who lived in an affluent community but struggled to make ends meet. When other parents went to the mall to buy new clothes, Donnie's parents went to the consignment store and bought the hand-me-downs of their neighbors. More than once as a young child, Donnie was miserably confronted and taunted by other children who recognized that he was wearing their old clothes. If this was not difficult enough for Donnie, he had other social obstacles. Living in a community in which looks and style were critical to popularity, Donnie was pathetically homely. His ears stuck out from his round face and his hair went every way but straight. He had not even the salvation of having some type of gift or talent. Rather, he was a slow learner, generally far behind his peers. However, to make matters worse for Donnie, he was not far enough behind to be placed in special classes. As a result, he, and his peers, simply saw him as stupid.

Donnie struggled through until high school. Someone—a school counselor, most probably—suggested to his parents that getting a job might help his self-esteem and self-confidence. It was arranged that Donnie interview to be a stockboy at the local grocery store. This could have worked out well except for two reasons. First, Donnie's lack of social abilities resulted in the same alienation and separation he experienced at school. Rather than being a social outcast just at school, he suffered the same indignities at the grocery store. None of the other kids would talk to him or even acknowledge him during breaks. His supervisor generally ignored him. Second, the grocery store was located in the same shopping center as the trendy stores frequented by his high school classmates. So, not only would they make fun of him or, worse, ignore him at school, they had now the additional opportunity of doing so while he worked.

Angry and alone, Donnie desperately wanted to gain some recognition, some achievement. He developed the idea that if a fire would break out in the store, he could be the first to spot it and rush all the people out. He would no longer be an outcast but a hero. Donnie dreamed and dreamed of this fantasy as he worked and suffered the taunts of his peers as they walked by. Trouble was, there never was a fire. So Donnie set one. Donnie, as in much of everything else, lacked knowledge of fires. The fire he set in the storeroom quickly leapt across the suspended ceiling, and soon the entire store was afire. Donnie barely escaped with his life and had no time to be a hero. Three people died in the fire. Donnie was convicted and sent to the juvenile correctional authority until he turned twenty-one.

Because fire can be very destructive, some children learn that setting fires is an excellent way to cover their tracks. They can either destroy the evidence of their misdeeds with the fire or simply draw attention away.

Just as the case with hurting animals, not all children who play with fire are potential antisocial personalities. Interest in fire appears to be a normal and natural part of development that responsible parents carefully direct and supervise. This interest in fire is termed *fire play*. The deliberate setting of fires for either control over others or to avoid responsibility is termed *fire setting*. A third and much more rare form of fire setting has been called *pyromania* and is seen in certain adolescents and adults who obtain sexual gratification through watching fires. Although this is perhaps the most commonly thought of explanation by most people for fire setting, it is, in fact, the most rare.

Chapter 3

Influences on Anger

THE DEVELOPMENT OF ANGER

Frankly, some children are just born difficult. It has nothing to do with how they are raised or how they have been treated. (Although, of course, problems in these areas can and do lead to later serious problems.) But most of the children who are "difficult" really don't want to be that way. They simply have brain organization and chemistry that makes them that way. This doesn't make them mentally ill or sick. They are more normal than abnormal. But they are different in how they react to the world, in how they show their feelings, and in their ability to control negative emotions. Because they are children, they are growing and pass through the same developmental stages as children who do not have difficult temperaments. For children who are irritable, angry, and difficult, their passage through these stages is different and often much more challenging for them and for their families, peers, and teachers.

In regard to how such children act during each stage of development, it is essential to keep in mind a few basic facts. First of all, although difficult children are more normal than not, without early intervention they are at much greater risk for later emotional and behavioral problems. With appropriate intervention, these children can and do lead lives that are healthy and meaningful. Because the inborn tendencies do not go away, however, they will always face challenges. They and the people around them will need to learn specific strategies and accommodations.

Second, no child chooses to be difficult. That is simply impossible. As discussed earlier, infants are born with different temperaments. Temperament is the internal, biological style of emotions and behaviors. It is but one part of personality. Overall, the personality is determined by the combination of what the child's biological makeup is at birth and the influences that come from the social environment. This is the classic "nature versus nurture" argument that has long been debated. The answer simply is that a child's personality results from the *interaction* between the inborn characteristics (nature) and the environment (nurture) of that child. Throughout the years, various movements have alternatively emphasized either one or the other. But the development of a child's personality is far more complex than a simple either/or. In some extreme cases, biological factors hold far more influence. In others, environmental factors are the greatest contributors to an individual's personality.

Developmental scientists have recently given proper focus to biological influences. For many years, the angry and difficult child was either blamed for his or her own behaviors or his or her parents were condemned as somehow failing to properly raise the child. But this is, at its face, simply implausible. Many infants, from the time of their birth, are fussy, colicky, difficult to soothe, difficult to get to sleep, and otherwise exhausting to the caregiver. How can that be the choice of the infants? They are developmentally unable to make such decisions. But often, temperamentally difficult children make their parents feel incompetent, inadequate, and at fault. The parents feel that the children won't listen to them, that they control them, and that nothing works. Parents blame themselves even when they are raising another child who has none of the difficult characteristics of the problem child. Can two children, raised by the same two parents, be so different only on the basis of parenting? Rarely. More likely than not, the difference is due to the interaction of the difficult personality of the infant and the parent's response (positive or negative) to that child.

The angry and difficult child is very tough and challenging to raise. What works for other children does not work for him or her. That is not to say that raising such a child is always an ordeal. Nor is it to say that the child will never change. Difficult children can have moments when they are wonderfully enjoyable. They can and do learn to regulate their tempers. But it is vital for parents who have an angry and difficult child to keep things in perspective. This problem is neither the fault of the child nor of the parents: it just simply is there. The sooner the parents can stop blaming themselves or their child, the more likely they can move on to learn ways to manage the child successfully. Through this different view, they can learn that one of the most important parental tasks that they face is teaching the child to manage his or her temper. This is not done through guilt, shame, and punishment. Rather, it is accomplished first by accepting that the task is difficult, that the child does want to do better, that there are specific skills that need to be gained, and that parents cannot accomplish this all by themselves. Most important, it is accomplished by building on the strengths of the child. This maxim holds not only for parents but also for all of the professionals that will encounter him or her.

What makes temperament? The study of temperament has most of its current scientific roots in the landmark New York Longitudinal Study by Alexander Thomas and colleagues. This study, begun in 1956, followed 133 persons from infancy to adulthood and focused upon the individuals' temperaments. It found that temperament differences were seen at birth, most clearly seen by eighteen months, and firmly established by the age of three. Differences in temperament are seen by measures of how active the child is; how impulsive the child is; how intense the child is with emotions; how predictable the child is with patterns of eating, sleep, and elimination; how persistent he or she is; how sensitive to stimuli in the environment; how does he or she respond to differing situations; how adaptable the child is; and what is his or her general disposition.

The easy-temperament child is not hyperactive and shows good self-control. In contrast, the difficult child always seems active and later is very impulsive. The easy child seems "mellow" and able to control his or her emotions. The difficult child is edgy, intense, and often intrusive with his or her moods. The easy child follows a schedule. The difficult child destroys it. The easy child tolerates changes and can adapt quickly to new sounds, new stimuli. The difficult child is rigid and inflexible and is prone to overreaction to new stimuli. The easy child seems to be basically cheerful, happy, and self-assured. The difficult child is nervous, intense, moody, and easily angered.

Difficult and angry children run along a continuum, a range. Some children simply have their moments but are able to pull together fairly quickly. At the other end, some children are so negative and difficult that they seem impossible to parent. Much of this can be the result of inborn characteristics, but much is not. Rather, the behavior of the child influences the behavior of the parent, which then influences the child. In the case of a difficult and angry child, it is easy for parents to find themselves trapped in a vicious circle that leads to frustration, anger, and giving up. Although it is very true that some angry and difficult children are "born that way," it is also very true that there is much that parents can do to bring about positive change.

In many ways, it is no different than any other parent whose child is born with a developmental challenge. Does the parent of a child born with a cleft palate simply give up and do nothing? Hardly. They brace themselves for the long and necessary ordeals of surgery and therapy that will eventually result in a normal or near-normal life for their child. Parents of a child who is born without sight don't simply allow their child to become dependent upon the sighted world for survival. They adapt and teach their child to adapt. The challenges faced by parents of difficult children are no different, and the hopes and expectations can be the same. Unfortunately, the disabilities faced by these children are terribly misunderstood. In a sad way, it would be easier for these children and their parents if they had been born with a visible disability. At least no one would be blamed. As much as I would like, I doubt if I will ever see a telethon or fund-raiser for difficult and angry children and their families.

A key aspect to the understanding of anger in children is understanding their patterns of social and language development. In early childhood, a young person first must establish basic relationships with the world around him or her and the people that fill that world. If care is provided in a consistent and predictable manner, then the child learns to trust that the world is a safe place. If, however, the child does not experience the world in that manner, or perhaps due to inborn temperament characteristics is unable to do so, he or she learns that the world is a place to be mistrusted. In this way, a basic pattern of interaction is established in which the child learns either to feel safe and comfortable or to be anxious and fearful, and, if required, learns to strike first in defense.

After about eighteen months and through age three, a child begins to decide whether he or she is competent or incompetent as a functioning person in the world. Although a bit clichéd, the time of interaction around toilet training is a critical time. If the child is able to successfully learn to control his or her eliminations, he or she succeeds in pleasing his or her parents. This is also the case with other major developmental tasks such as walking and talking. If the parents respond to his or her efforts in a positive manner, then the child gains a sense of success. The child will develop either feelings of autonomy or shame and doubt, depending upon whether he or she is able to accomplish these tasks and whether the parents react in a supportive manner or are harsh and critical. These feelings can form the beginnings of lifelong sadness and anger.

Between the ages of four and six, the child begins to expand his or her social horizons. The child begins to interact with others outside of the immediate family. He or she begins to be better able to complete tasks and often makes things or performs for significant adults, family members, or peers. If the child takes too much initiative, then he or she may grow up to be an overly forceful person who can become verbally or even physically aggressive. Conversely, the child may feel inadequate, insecure, and guilty if his or her efforts are unsuccessful or if the intended recipients are disparaging and rejecting. These experiences, as well, can lead to long-term feelings of inadequacy, depression, and anger.

Between the ages of seven and twelve, the child begins to move even farther out in the world (e.g., going to school). Here, the child must contend with the demands of others who are not in the family and who may not be as supportive. He or she is confronted with the need to learn new and increasingly complicated tasks. The success or failure of these experiences will result in a child feeling either that he or she is a person who has a sense of industry or competence or is an unsuccessful, inferior person. If a child begins to fall behind peers or is socially rejected because of his or her inadequacies, that child is likely to become a depressed, angry, and potentially isolated young person.

During adolescence, from the ages of thirteen to eighteen, the focus of the young person moves even farther out into the world. The young person begins to define himself or herself in the manner in which he or she relates to others. The young person needs to achieve a sense of identity in important areas such as occupation, social relationships, gender roles, spirituality, and achievement. If the adolescent is relatively successful in these areas, then he or she is able to develop a strong sense of personal identity. However, if the youth is unable to sort such matters out and is unsuccessful in obtaining a positive sense of self, a sense of role confusion will result. This role confusion can lead to further alienation, anger, and depression, which can alter the person's path through the rest of his or her life.

MEDIA AND THE DEVELOPMENT OF VIOLENCE

The effect of a young person's exposure to violence in the media cannot be minimized. Exposure to violence is pervasive in television, movies, music, and video games. The link between this exposure and violence is well established as a matter of scientific fact. According to the American Psychological Association (2001), today, over half of America's children have a television set in their bedrooms and they spend more time learning about life through mass media than through any other means. Before the age of eighteen, the average child in America will witness over 200,000 acts of violence on television alone, including over 16,000 murders. International studies have shown that the rate of homicides has doubled since the introduction of television to the country, even accounting for the introduction of television at differing times. Television and other media violence appear to have a stronger effect upon boys. Eight-year-old boys who viewed more violent programs growing up were the most likely to engage in aggressive and delinquent behavior by the age of eighteen and serious criminal behavior by the age of thirty. Although this research is newer, the exposure of children to violence through the Internet and through video games results in similar findings (Villani, 2001). This is not surprising in that much of the technology used to create popular violence-oriented video games results from the use of training methods developed by the military. The same findings hold true in reference to music. According to the surgeon general (Satcher, 1999b), the average American teenager listens to over 10,500 hours of music between seventh and twelfth grades, only about 500 hours less than they spend in school.

Chapter 4

Responses to Anger

Not all anger hurts. Actually, psychologists recognize that anger is a basic and essential human emotion. At times in all of our lives, it is appropriate to be angry. It is not so much the feeling of anger that may result in trouble. Rather, it is how we respond to that anger that can cause difficulty.

John

John worked out all summer to make the football team. He was new to the school, but not to football. In his previous school, he had been a wide receiver. Even though he had been just a freshman, he had gotten some playing time in the varsity games and had expected to make first string the next season. Then his father lost his job and the family was forced to move to another city so that his dad could find work. This new school was much larger than John's previous one. His sophomore class alone was larger than the entire high school that he had attended the year before. The school also had a long tradition of excelling in football. Numerous state championship trophies were in the high school display wall and many of the former players had gone on to college and even professional ranks as players. John never even made the first cut at the tryouts. He was beaten out by boys who were larger, faster, and stronger and who had played in that school system before. The day of tryouts, he had tried his best. The next day, when the list of players was posted, his name was not there. Angrily, he kicked the cement wall of the locker room and walked dejectedly off. Not easily stymied, he spent the next year working with weights, running, and attending a football camp run by one of the high school coaches. As a junior, he made the team. He never started but worked as hard as he could in practice, often playing on the "scout" team, allowing the first-string players the chance to practice against the plays of the upcoming opponents. At the end of the season, at the awards banquet, his parents proudly heard his coach praise John for not giving up and for channeling his anger at being cut the first year into the training that allowed him to make the team the next year.

John made choices. In this case, he made a responsible, productive one that eventually allowed him to achieve a goal originally denied him. John could have vented his anger in other, negative ways. He could have vandalized the stadium or taken his anger out on the family dog. He could have tried to smother his anger with alcohol and other drugs. Instead, he directed and focused his anger. There are many reasons why a person responds one way to anger and disappointment and another responds in a totally different manner. These reasons form the cornerstone of anger management with children and adolescents.

THE REACTION OF ANGER

Anger is a response. Most often, it is a response to what has happened to us in our world, our environment. Anger can be one reaction to the stress that we face in our lives. When we feel overwhelmed, kept from doing what we want to do, or pressed beyond our resources, it is only natural to respond emotionally. For children, the choice of emotion depends upon how they view or perceive the situation and, very important, what they have learned from past experiences and the experiences of others.

Stress can be positive or negative. Positive stressors can include getting married, having a child, getting a promotion at work, or buying a house. Negative stressors can include divorce, the death of a loved one, or financial misfortune. When we experience these events, our bodies respond in a genetically preprogrammed manner. Once a stressor is experienced, our brain activates our glandular system to send out certain chemical messengers to various parts of our bodies. This is the "fight-or-flight" reaction that can be best understood when we think of what happens when we corner an animal such as a dog or a cat. The animal first might attempt to run away. But, finding itself trapped, it will likely snarl, growl, raise the hair along its back, and signal that it is ready to fight.

Our genetic programming is really not all that different. In fact, we respond in much the same manner. When we are under stress certain things happen as a result of the chemical messengers sent out by certain glands such as the adrenals. Our heart beats faster; we breathe more rapidly; and the blood vessels in our hands and feet get smaller, forcing most of the blood to the internal organs (which is why we get cold hands and feet when we are nervous). In short, we become primed to fight. Because of this, our bodies remain keyed up and ready to fight. If we stay in a state of stress response for a long period of time, we can do considerable damage to our bodies and our emotions. For example, prolonged stress can increase vulnerability to disease and decrease the body's ability to fight it. We know that chronic stress can result in heart difficulties. In short, the link between psychological stress and physical illness has been long established. Managing stress is now a recognized and important aspect of health care.

Chronically time-conscious and hostile individuals ("type A personalities") have been shown to be at far greater risk of heart attack. Such persons are easily spotted in places such as the freeway. They speed down the road, tailgating, honking the horn while simultaneously shaving and talking on a cell phone. When we see such persons on the road (easily noticeable because of both the honking of the horns and the reflexive obscene gesture), it seems that some of them were likely even born with the middle finger raised in the air: "Jeez, Mom, what took you so long? Nine months? Give me a break! I have stock options to purchase, an IPO to research! And you, Doc! Could you warm up your hands a bit? Where's your fax machine? Because of your molasses-like delivery I have probably already lost out on the best deal of my young life!"

This scene might be a bit of a stretch, but chronic anger problems can most certainly impact the health of children. After all, the effects of anger and stress are not isolated to just adults. Although certain health problems such as cardiac disease may show cumulative effects, the effects upon the immune system are not. We know that chronically stressed children are more vulnerable to infections and disease. And we know that type A personalities don't just emerge at age thirty-five. They develop over time. Teaching the angry child to manage his or her anger has both long- and short-term benefits for you and the child.

RESILIENCE

In many people, anger can serve as a positive motivation to change. One of the more important concepts to understand in this dimension is that of resiliency. *Resilience* is the ability to bounce back, to recover from adverse circumstances. Resilience is also the ability to learn from adverse experiences and apply them to future difficulties.

A number of researchers, whose work is summarized by the surgeon general (Satcher, 1999b), have completed longitudinal-development studies of large groups of children growing up in various communities. Tracking these children through their development, researchers were able to identify risk and protective factors that served to either make a child more vulnerable or resistant to problems. The concept of resiliency theory is that we have learned much about what we know of children through the studies of children who have had problems. Very little is known about the qualities of those children who faced similar circumstances and triumphed instead of being defeated. These factors, termed protective factors, are those features that serve to protect the child against the poor outcomes that are usually associated with risk factors. Typical risk factors that are studied include fetal drug or alcohol effects, premature birth or complications, a difficult temperament, a shy temperament, neurological impairment and low IQ, a chronic medical disorder, mental illness of either the child or the parents, repeated aggression against the child or exposure to repeated aggression against others, substance abuse by the child or others responsible for the care of that child, and delinquent or antisocial behavior by the child or those responsible for the care of the child.

These factors, of course, are well known and well documented. Less well known are the qualities of a resilient person. Research shows that certain protective factors do insulate a child. These factors include being born with an easy temperament, autonomy and independence as a toddler, high hopes and expectations for the future, a sense of good personal identity and self-confidence as an adolescent, good interpersonal skills resulting in being a "likeable person," a sense of humor, empathy for others, perceiving oneself as competent and capable, having an average or above-average IQ, being a good reader, relating well to others, and having good problem-solving skills.

Some of these characteristics cannot be be changed. Although IQ is not a fixed number and can be modified through education and experience, such changes are typically limited to a certain range. Thus, although a person may be intellectually below average due to early childhood deprivation, some aspects of IQ (e.g., the influence of poor prenatal nutrition and substance abuse) are less easily overcome. But many of the qualities of resiliency can be taught or acquired. Recall from Chapter 2 that development was discussed through the model of Piaget. These developmental stages provide clear opportunities to engage a child in a positive manner that builds protective factors. Much of these capacities are gained through positive adults. If parents are not available or capable of providing these qualities, then the use of other caring adults as "mentors" can produce many beneficial results.

Chapter 5

Anger and Emotional Problems

Most children who struggle with anger problems are not seriously disturbed in their ability to relate to others. They want to be connected but act in a manner that prevents or limits that very thing. As much as we would like to try, children don't fall into neat categories. Often, the problem of anger coexists with other problems. The most typical problems are ADHD, oppositional defiant disorder (ODD), depression, substance abuse, and conduct disorder. Each of these disorders can result in considerable problems with anger as well as causing significant distress in both the family and at school.

This chapter will present information on these disorders. It is important to note, however, that this discussion is not a substitute for a comprehensive evaluation by a qualified mental health professional. If your child does seem to fit one or more of the problem areas described, you should seek advice from a qualified mental health professional, your pediatrician, school counselor, or local mental health agency. Many resources are available and a considerable number provide services with a sliding scale of fees.

ATTENTION-DEFICIT HYPERACTIVITY DISORDER

Attention-deficit hyperactivity disorder (ADHD) is one of the most common and most frequently misunderstood diagnoses of children and adolescents. It is a real disorder that causes real problems, both for the person who has that disorder as well as the persons who live with or interact with that person. ADHD is surrounded by myth and misunderstanding. It is a genuine condition, most probably due to abnormalities in brain chemistry and structure. It is not due to poor parenting, laziness, or simple unwillingness. A popular opinion is that ADHD is overdiagnosed and a rationalization for control of "normal" child behavior through medication. In fact, research shows conclusively that untreated persons with ADHD are at far greater risk for other problems and disorders, including substance abuse, than are those who are successfully treated with a combination of behavioral therapy and medication.

Currently, the best source for understanding of and resources for ADHD is the organization known as Children and Adults with Attention-Deficit/Hyperactivity Disorder (CHADD). Their Web site <www.chadd.org> provides the most comprehensive and up-to-date information available on this disorder. If, after reading this section, you feel that your child suffers from ADHD, you are urged to contact either the national or a local chapter of CHADD.

Many children have difficulty sitting still, paying attention, or controlling impulsive behavior. However, for some, this difficulty is so pervasive and persistent that it interferes with their ability to live a happy and productive life.

ADHD is characterized by developmentally inappropriate impulsivity, attention, and, in some cases, hyperactivity. According to the American Academy of Child and Adolescent Psychiatry (1999), the present understanding of ADHD is that it is a neurobiological disorder that affects 3 to 5 percent of school-age children. Parenting does not cause it; however, ADHD can clearly result in family problems, which can contribute to parenting problems that make the behaviors worse rather than better. Researchers once thought that children with ADHD simply "grew out of it" after adolescence. Now we know differently. Current estimates are that at least 2 to 5 percent of the adult population suffers from ADHD. About 50 to 60 percent of children with ADHD will continue to experience symptoms into adulthood (Barkley, 1995). What does seem to go away, for many, is the hyperactive and impulsive part. Some researchers believe that adults simply learn to cope with and adapt to their impulsive urges. However, the problems with inattention, focus, concentration, and distractibility often do not go away. In fact, these problems can often cause significant distress in adults who see themselves (or are seen by others) as having negative personal characteristics. However, in reality, they suffer from unrecognized ADHD. It is estimated by the National Institute of Mental Health (1996) that approximately 20 million children and adults suffer from ADHD.

There is no reason that a person with ADHD who is successfully treated cannot lead a productive and meaningful life. In fact, many creative and accomplished people have ADHD. Untreated, ADHD can lead to serious problems with conduct, depression, social failure, educational failure, and poor job performance in later life. A common fear is that treatment of ADHD with stimulant medication will increase the child's vulnerability to substance abuse. In fact, the opposite is true. Children who have ADHD and who are *not* treated are at the greatest risk.

The symptoms common to ADHD have been recognized since the beginning of the twentieth century. Since that time, ADHD has had many names, a problem that has contributed to the misunderstanding of this disorder. Names once used for the syndrome include minimal brain dysfunction, hyperkinetic reaction of childhood, and attention-deficit disorder with or without hyperactivity. With the publication of the latest manual for diagnosis of psychological problems, the *Diagnostic and Statistical Manual of Mental Disorders,* Fourth Edition, Text Revision, in 2000, the diagnostic understanding of ADHD was significantly changed to attention-deficit hyperactivity disorder, hyperactive-impulsive type; attention-deficit hyperactivity disorder, predominately inattentive type; and attention-deficit disorder, combined type. This reclassification was made to recognize the importance of attention problems in each of the various subtypes.

Children who have problems mostly with being hyperactive and impulsive and not so much with attention or concentration are typically diagnosed with attention-deficit hyperactivity disorder, hyperactive-impulsive type. This is the category most often described as "hyper" and is often what most people think of as ADHD. At the other end of the continuum, children who have the opposite pattern are seen as attention-deficit hyperactivity disorder, predominately inattentive type. These children do not usually behave in a manner that is impulsive or hyperactive. They often seem to be daydreaming, forgetful, and disorganized. Sometimes when parents of these children are told that their child suffers from ADHD, they are confused because of the lack of hyperactive behavior. Some may disagree and say that they see ADD, which is what was then the understanding and name of this subtype. Last, children who show both types of problems are given the diagnosis of attention-deficit hyperactivity disorder, combined type. These children typically are first seen during their preschool years, being mostly hyperactive. As they grow older, often after entering formal schooling, they begin to show additional problems with attention, focus, organization, and memory. Not all researchers support that these three types are homogenous. One fact pointed out is that children with the predominately inattentive type of ADHD are much less likely to develop behavioral and conduct problems than those children who are seen as hyperactive-impulsive or combined. When inattentive ADHD children do develop problems, they seem to be related more to depression, anxiety, and poor self-esteem. That is, they tend to internalize and the hyperactive type tends to externalize their problems.

ADHD is believed to be the result of a biochemical imbalance in specific parts of the brain, and increasing evidence using magnetic resonance imaging (MRI) has been able to suggest differences in brain formation, primarily in the frontal lobes (especially the left) that are responsible for the "executive functions" of the brain, such as planning, organization, sustained concentration, judgment, and impulse control. Some types of ADHD-like symptoms are the result of injury to the brain, toxins (such as the ingestion of lead), or perinatal insult (such as substance abuse while pregnant). ADHD is not related to intelligence. Many persons with ADHD are bright, even gifted and creative thinkers. However, ADHD is related to difficulties in learning as a result of problems paying attention and hyperactivity. Russell Barkley (1995) estimated that about 30 percent of children with ADHD do suffer from some sort of learning disability. Although it is thought that ADHD is far more common in boys, Phelan (1996) suggests that ADHD appears equally often in girls but may go unrecognized.

ADHD has certain major characteristics. The first is that of impaired response inhibition, impulse control, or difficulties in delaying gratification. Often, ADHD children will stand out as those who are unable to stop and think before acting, who have trouble waiting for their turn in line, who often interrupt others, who prefer short-term rewards over long-term goals, and who have extreme difficulty not being distracted. Second, ADHD youth frequently are seen as being involved in behaviors or activities that are not related to the task at hand. They may always seem to be on the go, and are typically described by parents as driven by a motor. In situations such as school, they show excessive movement such as fidgeting, tapping, wiggling feet or hands, rocking, or just not being able to sit still. Younger children may not be able to sit still at all and often show excessive motor activities such as climbing, running, etc. Even though this does decrease with age, teenagers with ADHD tend to be more restless than other teens. Adults, as well, even though they may not be outwardly as hyperactive, do report that they often feel restless and need to stay busy and have trouble sitting still for any length of time. A third characteristic is that of significant difficulty paying attention or sticking with tasks. This is especially seen when they have to do something that is boring or repetitious. In such circumstances, when compared to other people, they seem to be less persistent and have trouble sticking with the task. Often this can be misunderstood as a lack of motivation or even laziness.

Again, following the model of Barkley (1995), ADHD youth, particularly those who are hyperactive and impulsive, often have certain psychological characteristics in addition to the behavioral problems noted previously. They often have trouble with memory, tend to be forgetful, and are unable to keep important information in mind. Parents of ADHD children often are totally frustrated when not only do the children forget to bring home homework, sometimes they will forget to even turn it in when they go back to school. Adults with ADHD are forever losing their keys, cell phones, and even handheld planners. They sometimes lose track of the goal of their initial activity because they have gotten distracted by something or more than one thing. They have considerable difficulty with time management and are often late.

ADHD youth are often behind in the development of "self-talk" or the internal language of thinking. We all have private voices inside our heads that guide and direct our behavior. Research indicates that ADHD youth are delayed in this development when compared to non-ADHD youth. This ability is important for individuals to be able to follow through on their own plans, create "to-do" lists, or even act with rules, legal imperatives, or moral principles in mind. In school, ADHD youth often have trouble with reading comprehension, especially long, complex, and boring assignments due to the combination of delay in internal language development and problems with working memory.

ADHD youth are also delayed in their ability to control their emotions, their motivations, and their level of arousal. They appear to be socially immature and are often much less able to keep their thoughts and feelings to themselves. They may blurt things out that may offend others or embarrass their parents without realizing what they are doing. They often tend to have anger control problems and impulsively act upon negative feelings, which is why this discussion is so important to understanding an angry child. They, as well, often seem to be daydreaming, be lost in their own world, and have difficulty with self-motivation.

Children with ADHD often have very poor problem-solving abilities, both practically and socially. They tend to be repetitive in how they approach a problem, even if they have tried that solution before and it has failed. As well, they tend to give up easily on tasks that seem difficult for them and seem to be less creative at finding new ways to approach an old problem. Even in their writing and spoken words, they seem to have trouble organizing their thoughts or responding appropriately to questions.

A final psychological characteristic of ADHD is that of considerable variability in how they are able to do things. They often show, much to the consternation and confusion of others, wide swings in their ability to successfully complete tasks. Frustrated parents often cannot understand why their ADHD children were able to complete their mathematics homework quickly and accurately just the night before and the next time do completely the opposite.

ADHD shows itself early in life, on the average between the ages of three to six years. But, as might be expected with ADHD children, not all fall neatly within these time frames. Some ADHD children do not show symptoms until somewhat later, often when schoolwork becomes more demanding and the days are longer. Most certainly, however, the majority of ADHD children have had some symptoms before the age of thirteen. One characteristic of ADHD that leads to frequent misunderstanding and mislabeling is that ADHD symptoms are not always consistent. ADHD children are very sensitive to changes in their environments and often do much better in one-to-one situations. Again, the frustrated parent may ask, "Why could you do that with me and then not in class?" They often behave much better when the tasks are specific, are broken down into small parts, and have immediate rewards.

People do not grow out of ADHD. Years ago, it was thought that ADHD symptoms often went away, especially after puberty. Recent research using better methods and criteria has found that this is not the case at all. Rather, less than 30 percent of children with ADHD outgrow their symptoms (Barkley, 1998). Although most ADHD children do not have serious problems in other areas, the fact remains that ADHD children are more at risk for other social, behavioral, and emotional problems as adolescents and adults. Barkley (1998) also reports that about one-quarter of children diagnosed with ADHD also meet the DSM-IV diagnostic criteria for conduct disorder and about one-third meet the diagnostic criteria for oppositional defiant disorder. About 10 percent develop bipolar disorder and between 10 and 20 percent go on to develop an antisocial personality in adulthood. About 10 to 25 percent develop problems with substance abuse and tobacco use. Although these statistics seem dismal, it is important to remember that 50 percent of ADHD children *do not* develop these problems. Many who do have those problems are also children who are exposed to considerable psychosocial stressors such as loss of a parent, frequent moving, and other factors. Yet the vast majority of children with ADHD do experience problems with education and require specialized intervention if they are to succeed academically and vocationally.

Sammy

The staff at the residential treatment center defined Sammy as the "ADHD poster child." He was constantly on the go, except when he had to do his homework. Then he would shut down, sullenly stare at the paper, and suddenly, in a nanosecond, be squirming around in his chair, imitating noises of bodily functions, and throwing spitballs. Sammy, however, entered the Hall of Fame one day while the board of trustees of the treatment center was meeting. Shortly after the usual presentations by the agency's executive director and the clinical director, one of the lights in the suspended ceiling began to shake, catching the eye of a few board members. All of them, however, did notice Sammy as he fell through the ceiling and landed on the conference table.

The Diagnosis of ADHD

Because almost all children show some ADHD-like behaviors at one time or another, specific and careful diagnosis is required. As stated by CHADD, to be diagnosed with ADHD, individuals must exhibit a minimum of six characteristics in either or both of two

DSM-IV categories, which include a list of nine characteristics of inattention and nine characteristics of hyperactivity or impulsivity. In children and teenagers, the symptoms must be more frequent or severe than in other children the same age. In adults, the symptoms must affect the ability to function in daily life and persist from childhood. In addition, the behaviors must create significant difficulty in at least two areas of life, such as home, social settings, school, or work. Symptoms must be present for at least six months.

How Should the Child Be Evaluated?

There is no specific test for ADHD. Diagnosis is a multifaceted process that involves multiple observations over time. ADHD can be confused with many other problems, as many biological and psychological problems can contribute to symptoms similar to those exhibited by children with ADHD. Children who are depressed, anxious, and have a history of abuse may resemble ADHD children at first glance. To simply say that a child has ADHD because he or she is hyperactive or inattentive is not acceptable. Because of this, an ADHD evaluation needs to be comprehensive. A careful history must be taken and observations from multiple observers of the child in multiple settings should be obtained. Most typically, these observations should be obtained by using a well-researched, standardized rating scale. If the child has not had a medical examination, this should be the first priority. Several types of professionals can diagnose ADHD, including school psychologists, private psychologists, social workers, nurse practitioners, neurologists, psychiatrists, and other medical doctors. Regardless of who does the evaluation, the use of DSM-IV-TR criteria is necessary. A medical exam by a physician is important and should include a thorough physical examination, including hearing and vision tests, to rule out other medical problems that may be causing symptoms similar to ADHD. In rare cases, persons with ADHD also may have a thyroid dysfunction. Only medical doctors as well as nurse practitioners and psychologists in certain states and settings can prescribe medication if it is needed.

Treatment of ADHD

There is no cure for ADHD. Rather, treatments manage and control symptoms and build new skills. For treatment to be effective, it must be multimodal and build on the strengths of the child and his or her family. Multimodal means that a variety of interventions in the home and in the school, possibly medication, as well as individual counseling is likely required. The research on treatment outcome, especially the NIMH Multimodal Treatment Study of ADHD, is very encouraging. Children who received medication alone or in combination with behavioral treatment showed significant improvement in their behavior and academic work as well as better relationships with their classmates and family.

Primary among treatments that are successfully used is the combination of behavioral management, cognitive-behavioral therapy, and psychostimulant medications such as methylphenidate (Ritalin), amphetamines, or amphetamine combinations (Dexedrine and Adderall). Approximately 70 to 80 percent of children with ADHD respond positively to psychostimulant medications. Significant academic improvement is shown by students who take these medications: *increased* attention and concentration, compliance and effort on tasks, and amount and accuracy of schoolwork produced; and *decreased* activity levels, impulsivity, negative behaviors in social interactions, and physical and verbal interchanges. Some children will respond better to differing types of medications (e.g., antidepressants, such as Wellbutrin [bupropion hydrochloride]). Many of these medications have introduced longer-acting versions. Recently, a nonstimulant medication, Strattera (amoxetine HCL), was approved by the FDA for the treatment of ADHD. Strattera differs from other medications because it is a selective norepinephrine reuptake inhibitor.

In the area of psychological treatments, the most effective are those that focus on parent education and training and modifications in the classroom. Behavioral techniques are generally positive reinforcement (or reward-based) systems in which a child gains points or privileges for desired behavior. It is important to note two things about behavioral treatment. First of all, the research suggests that ADHD children who are treated only with behavioral methods and not medication are likely to show only short-term benefits. In studies where medication was used then discontinued, it was found that the behavioral treatment alone was not effective. ADHD children often require specific training in skills such as time management, planning lists, and social skills. In schools, children with ADHD may be eligible for special educational services under both the Individuals with

Disabilities in Education Act (IDEA) and Section 504 of the Rehabilitation Act of 1973. When a parent suspects that his or her child does have ADHD, the parent should contact the school and request a multifactored evaluation (MFE). Schools that tell parents that only children with specific learning disabilities are eligible for an MFE and the subsequent individualized education plan or a 504 Plan should be reminded of the two previously noted federal laws. In the case of adults, if ADHD produces serious impairment in one or more areas of life functioning and is disclosed to the employer, persons with ADHD are also eligible for accommodations under the Americans with Disabilities Act, provided that it can be shown that the disability does produce sufficient functional impairment at the work site.

Some treatments for ADHD have little or no evidence of any effectiveness. Primary of these are dietary management techniques, such as the removal of sugar from the diet. As well, megavitamin therapy, minerals, trace elements, or other popular health food remedies have been shown to be ineffective. Long-term therapy, psychoanalysis, biofeedback, play therapy, chiropractic treatment, or sensory-integration approaches have not proven to be effective in the treatment of ADHD.

OPPOSITIONAL DEFIANT DISORDER

As previously mentioned, 30 to 50 percent of children with ADHD, especially those with the combined and hyperactive-impulsive types, are at risk for developing more severe behavioral problems such as oppositional defiant disorder (ODD) and conduct disorder (Barkley, 1998). Again, as was the case with ADHD, careful, multifactored diagnoses of these conditions is required. It is part of normal development for children to be stubborn and at times negativistic. All children at some time or another will test limits. This is part of the development of a healthy individual personality. But there are those children, especially those with ADHD, whose degree of noncompliance becomes pervasive and problematic. The term *noncompliance* needs to be carefully used (Barkley, 1997), and includes failure of the child to respond in a reasonably timely manner to adult directions, failure to continue compliance with directions, and failure to follow previously learned rules of behavior in a situation. Noncompliance can be passive and resistant. Thus, a child may, on one hand, throw a substantial temper tantrum or, on the other hand, simply avoid or ignore parental or teacher directions.

Since some degree of oppositional and resistive behavior is normal, most authorities, such as Barkley (1997) and Green (1998) suggest that specific criteria must be used to determine if the child does suffer from ODD rather than simple noncompliance. Common throughout these criteria is the question of whether the oppositional behavior consistently impairs the child's effective functioning across differing situations. More specifically, the behavior of the child must be significantly different from his or her peers. Most of the time, this determination is made through the use of standardized rating scales that are completed by a variety of persons familiar with the child.

If a child misbehaves with only one person or in one setting, the problem is likely more situational-focused than ODD. When the child is seen as exhibiting a level of oppositional and defiant behavior that is beyond that usually expected for persons of that age, this criteria is not in and of itself sufficient. The child must also suffer a significant degree of adaptive impairment. Simply put, does the problem behavior significantly interfere with the child being able to meet the demands and realize the developmental capacities for a child that age? For example, when compared to other children, does the child care for himself or herself adequately; does he or she fulfill expected requirements such as homework and chores? Does he or she show age-appropriate interactions with peers and adults? Or is he or she so oppositional and defiant that such expectations are rarely if ever achieved? Do the oppositional and defiant behavior needs result in feelings of discomfort or even harm by either the child or the family and other significant adults?

Many of the children with ODD not only make people around them feel miserable, but they themselves feel miserable. They have poor self-concepts and see themselves as being inferior to other children. Even if the oppositional and defiant behaviors are beyond that usually expected, resulting in impairment and distress, it is important that these behaviors do not arise from other, missed problems. Children who are depressed, who are beginning to show signs of bipolar disorder, or who are being victimized and abused may show similar symptoms.

Jeffrey

If Sammy was the ADHD poster child to the residential treatment center staff, then Jeffrey was well on his way to achieving their award of oppositional defiance and hyperactivity with distinction. One staff member related that when she tried to redirect Jeffrey he became loud, profane, and angry in sharing his displeasure. He became so agitated that he literally climbed the wall, thus earning him the status of legend among the clinical staff. The staff did begin to notice a pattern with him, however. He was much worse on Mondays and then through the week seemed to actually improve. Since he went to a county children's services approved placement (his paternal grandfather) on the weekends, the staff supposed that much of his problem was due to having to readjust to the structure and expectations of the treatment center. Then, one Monday, Jeffrey set the residential cottage on fire. No one was hurt and the fire was put out fairly quickly with minimal damage. Jeffrey was transferred from the open cottage setting of the facility to the locked, secure unit. The staff interviewed him, and learned that each weekend Jeffrey went to his grandfather's house, he would be taken to the attic, shown pornographic movies, and sexually molested by his grandfather. The visits were terminated, the grandfather was prosecuted, and Jeffrey's hyperactivity and oppositional behavior melted away.

When a child truly has ODD, he or she is at greater risk for lifelong problems. About half will continue to show oppositional defiance throughout childhood and adolescence. Nearly half of these will develop a more serious conduct disorder, which involves actual delinquent behavior and physical aggression as well as substance abuse (Barkley, 1997). Thus, although not all children with ADHD will develop ODD, and not all children with ODD will progress to a conduct disorder, most of the children who do progress into conduct disorder do show symptoms of ODD. Thus, there appears to be a clear pathway for a certain percentage of children from ADHD to ODD and then to conduct disorder.

Diagnostic Criteria for ODD

In order to meet the DSM-IV criteria for ODD, the child must, as noted earlier, demonstrate a pattern of behavior that persists across time and situation and is not due to other problems. Further, the behavior must result in significant impairment in the child's ability to function at a developmentally appropriate level. The DSM-IV requires a persistent "pattern of negativistic, hostile, and defiant behavior toward authority figures that persists for at least 6 months and is characterized by the frequent occurrence of at least four of the following" behaviors (p. 91) (reprinted with permission from the *Diagnostic and Statistical Manual of Mental Disorders,* Fourth Edition. Copyright 1994, American Psychiatric Association). The child must demonstrate behaviors such as losing his or her temper, arguing with adults, actively defying or refusing to comply with the requests of others, deliberately annoying people, blaming others for his or her mistakes or misbehavior, being touchy and easily annoyed, being angry and resentful, and being spiteful or vindictive.

Causes of ODD

When studies are made of the families of ODD children, many but not all of them appear to have similar characteristics. The hallmark of these characteristics is that the parents are often harsh and inconsistent in how they discipline the children. They, as well, often have histories of poor monitoring of the children. They are generally so unpredictable that the children naturally seek to avoid interaction with the parents for fear of disproportionately negative consequences. However, it is not at all fair, or supported in the research, to say that parenting is the sole cause of ODD. Not only do ODD children have specific individual traits, but also the actions of the children influence the parents who then influence the actions of the children. Parenting is very much a reciprocal, give-and-take process and defiant children can significantly affect how their parents treat them. Conversely, it has been found that parents who are themselves immature, impulsive, oppositional, hostile, rejecting, negativistic, and defiant are more likely to produce children with ODD (Olweus, 1993; Patterson, Capaldi, and Bank, 1991).

One emerging trend in research concerning oppositional children is that of their temperament. Children with ODD were difficult as infants and were fussy and difficult to please. They were irregular in sleep and eating habits and generally very negative in mood. As older children, they are more inattentive and impulsive and easily angered. They often learn to control others through their negative behaviors. If untreated, males tend to show such behavior throughout later childhood and adolescence. For females, the presence of oppositional behavior as a young child is linked more to later problems with depression and anxiety than conduct problems. An important psychological aspect of ODD is the strong relationship between its diagnosis and ADHD, especially the hyperactive-impulsive and the combined types. In the section on ADHD, it was noted that nearly half of children with ADHD are at risk for ODD. It has been shown that the combination of poor impulse control, hyperactivity, and oppositionality at an early age is likely to emerge into very difficult problems in individual, family, and school functioning (Barkley, 1997).

Physical characteristics may also place a child at greater risk for ODD. At a very basic level, children with ODD tend to be much more sensitive to stimulation from their environments. They overreact to noises, changes in temperature and lighting, as well as the movement and activities of others. As young children, they cry easily and are often irritable. They have difficulty establishing regular habits in eating, elimination, and sleeping. ODD children respond much more negatively to demands placed upon them by schedules, often develop problems such as colic, or are picky eaters.

Their physical appearance, coordination, strength, stamina, and other abilities may also be critical factors in determining how they react to others. Children who are physically unattractive may become oppositional and defiant as a defense mechanism. That is, they act in a manner that rejects others first before others have a chance to reject them. When they act this way, they are generally more prone to being disliked and rejected by peers and adults, which then further leads to a lower self-image and more oppositional behavior. Sometimes children behave in an oppositional and defiant manner just to obtain attention from a parent or peers. For some children, negative attention is far better than positive. Some suffer simply because they look or act like someone with whom the adult has had previous negative experiences.

CONDUCT DISORDERS

Many of the children who suffer from ODD will progress to the most severe form of what the DSM-IV-TR terms disruptive behavioral disorders, conduct disorder (Barkley, 1997). This disorder, often a controversial disorder because of the seemingly circular definition, describes children and adolescents who show a persistent pattern of behavior that violates social norms and the rights of others. Conduct disorder is broken down into two primary types: childhood onset (before the age of ten) and adolescent onset (after the age of ten). Conduct disorder is also subdivided into levels of severity: mild, moderate, and severe.

Rick

Rick, a sixteen-year-old white male, was charged with one count of aggravated murder, aggravated robbery, aggravated burglary, and theft. He and another youth broke out of a state juvenile correctional facility and traveled to a nearby small town, which was the home of the other youth. They went to the house of an elderly man who had testified against the other youth, attacked and beat him, robbed his house, and kidnapped the victim by placing him in the trunk of his car. They then drove to a river and threw the victim off of a bridge. Although he was apparently alive when thrown from the bridge, the man died on impact.

At the time of forensic evaluation, Rick was in the lockup area of the correctional facility after attacking and threatening to kill a staff member. Records indicated that he was the second of four children from an extremely problematic childhood characterized by substance abuse, physical abuse, neglect, and instability. All of the children were in the care of various agencies and the family was described as highly resistant to treatment. Rick was diagnosed as hyperactive in the first grade and became involved in the juvenile justice system at age eight. His first out-of-home placement took place at age eleven. He was placed in juvenile correctional facilities at age twelve following an attempt to stab another youth. At age fourteen, Rick attempted to strangle a youth with a belt. His juvenile court record subsequently contained charges of attacks upon others, holding a knife to a child's throat, arson, and carrying a concealed weapon. Assaultive behavior, self-mutilation, escape, and suicidal threats characterized his institutional placement. Clinically, Rick was seen as ADHD and with severe conduct disorder. No evidence of psychosis was ever reported. Intellectually, Rick consistently presented within the borderline range of general intelligence.

In forensic evaluation, Rick reported an extensive history of being physically abused but denied being sexually abused. He reported an extensive history of substance abuse beginning at age nine. He described his temper control problems as, "I just flip; any little thing can make me mad. I just strike out." He was able to relate the details of the alleged offense, had a clear working knowledge of the justice system, and expressed an understanding of the attorney-youth relationship. On a standardized intelligence test, Rick was found to function within the borderline range of general intelligence with no significant advantage in verbal or performance skills. He had strengths in social awareness and basic visual motor reproduction skills. Difficulties were seen in tasks requiring abstractions of either a verbal or visual motor nature, and he had particular difficulty in tasks that required judgment. There was an indication of a learning disorder related to a limited attention span and visual perceptual processing difficulties. Psychological testing was not found to be indicative of psychosis but did suggest impulsivity, poor judgment, poor emotional control, and a view of interpersonal relationships as hostile and conflicted. Rick expressed no substantial regret for his actions, believing that the elderly victim had deserved his fate. Rick had also turned in the other youth with whom he had committed the crimes. Rick also indicated that he preferred to be placed in the adult system because he wanted to go to prison. He did state that he was aware that if he were placed in the juvenile system, he would be out sooner and stated that, if returned to the community, he would, "get busted again." Rick was assessed as not being amenable to further treatment in the juvenile justice system and was bound over to the adult court. He entered a plea of guilty to murder and received a sentence of twenty years to life, with a possibility of parole within seven years.

Diagnostic Criteria for Conduct Disorder

Youth with conduct disorder may exhibit some of the following characteristics. In order to meet the criteria for a conduct disorder, three or more of these behaviors must have been seen for at least twelve months and at least one must be present in the six months immediately prior to any diagnosis. They have a pattern of aggression to persons or animals in which they bully, threaten, or intimidate; often initiate physical fights; have used a weapon; have been physically cruel to persons or animals; have stolen from victims while confronting them (e.g., mugging or assault); or have forced someone into sexual activity. As well, they may have a pattern of destruction of property in which they may have deliberately engaged in fire setting with the intention to cause damage or deliberately destroyed the property of another. They also may have a pattern of deceitfulness, stealing, or lying in which they may have broken into someone else's house, building, or car; a pattern of lying to obtain goods or favors or to avoid obligations; or a pattern of stealing items without confronting the victim (e.g., shoplifting without breaking and entering). Last, they may evidence a pattern of serious violations of rules such as staying out late at night despite curfew or parental permission, running away from home at least twice or once without returning for a long period of time, and may often be truant from school beginning before the age of thirteen. It is important to note that these problems must cause a serious degree of impairment in the youth's adaptive functioning and are not the result of other emotional problems or social situations (reprinted with permission from the *Diagnostic and Statistical Manual of Mental Disorders,* Fourth Edition. Copyright 1994, American Psychiatric Association).

Youth with these behaviors obviously require a fairly intense evaluation. Many with conduct disorders are likely to have coexisting disorders such as mood disorders, severe anxiety, substance abuse, post-traumatic stress disorder, ADHD, learning problems, or serious mental illnesses, such as a psychosis.

Causes of Conduct Disorder

In recent years, a new understanding of antisocial and aggressive behaviors has emerged using a developmental pathway model. Much of this new view can be credited to the work of Gerald Patterson and his colleagues. Rather than viewing conduct problems as behaviors that suddenly happen or as a reaction to a circumstance, violence is seen as a pattern of behavior characteristic of the child. Antisocial and aggressive behavior is a pattern that emerges at an early age. Without intervention, antisocial behavior and violence remain an enduring characteristic of the person. It appears to be a developmental trait that begins early in life and often continues into adolescence and adulthood. For many youth, stable manifestations of antisocial behavior begin as early as prekindergarten ages.

A significant body of research by Patterson and his colleagues (1989) suggests an "early starter model," which describes a family matrix that directly trains youth in antisocial behavior. It is suggested that the family directly reinforces the aggressive and antisocial behavior of the child. These antisocial behaviors then transfer from the home to other settings and then lead to social failures. The end result of this process is an enduring pattern of antisocial and aggressive behavior. Patterson and his colleagues (1989) suggest that antisocial behavior seen at grade four is predictive of later aggressive behavior. A number of developmental variables have been consistently identified as covariates for aggression in both youth and adults. As indicated by Patterson and colleagues, families of aggressive youth are characterized by harsh and inconsistent discipline, and aggressive individuals are frequently the victims of physical abuse as children. Parents tend to be socially unskilled and inept, so that the child learns to manipulate or coerce others instead of learning appropriate social skills. Although some parents may positively reinforce aggressive behavior, escape/avoidance is often the primary factor; the child uses aversive behavior to terminate aversive intrusions by family members. He or she acts obnoxiously to force others to leave him or her alone. As the pattern continues, the parents escalate their coercion to hitting and physical attacks, and thus the child learns that aggression can be used to control others. This pattern of aggression leads to rejection by the peer group, not the reverse, and results in either deviant peer group membership or social isolation.

Rejected aggressive youth are deficient in a number of prosocial skills including positive peer group entry, perception of peer group norms, and response to provocation and interpretation of prosocial interactions. Family stresses such as substance abuse, poverty, divorce, and domestic violence are equally associated with violent youth. There is a high degree of intergenerational similarity for antisocial behavior. Having one antisocial, aggressive parent places a child at significant risk for aggressive behavior, with an even higher risk when both parents are antisocial. Patterson has documented concordance across three generations.

Quinn and colleagues (1995) found that critical factors identified those first-grade boys who were at risk for developing antisocial behavior. These factors were higher teacher ratings of aggression, more negative peer interactions on the playground, and lower levels of academic-engaged time compared to their peers. Stability coefficients for childhood aggression challenge those of intelligence quotients. Early behaviors such as temper tantrums and grade-school troublesomeness have been found to significantly predict youth and adult offenses, and suggest an underlying developmental continuum. Nursery school children who obtain goals through aggression are likely to go on using this behavior to pursue such goals. Longitudinal studies of both Swedish and American youth show a clear pattern of aggression beginning in preschool and continuing to adulthood. The studies reveal one group of chronically aggressive youth and another group of chronic victims. The aggressive behavior of the youth was consistent and evident as long as fifteen years later.

MOOD DISORDERS

Perhaps the most common and most frequently misunderstood and unrecognized problem in children and adolescents is the mood disorder. Generally, when we think of depression, we think of it in adult terms: crying, sadness, isolation, and withdrawal. Although many children who do suffer from a mood disorder can be like that, many who suffer from a mood disorder are just the opposite. It is quite likely that a child who suffers from a mood disorder may act out his or her problems in ways that are oppositional, defiant, and sometimes delinquent.

The U.S. surgeon general, in his document "Mental Health: A Report of the Surgeon General" (Satcher, 1999a), estimated that at any one time between 10 and 15 percent of the child and adolescent population of the United States suffers from some symptoms of depression. As detailed in the surgeon general's report, the prevalence of the diagnosis of full-fledged major depression between the ages of nine and seventeen is estimated to be 5 percent and the prevalence of the chronic but less acute dysthymic disorder is estimated to be around 3 percent. Taken together, these statistics indicate that many of our youth suffer in significant ways from depression. Beyond that, suicide among children and adolescents remains a serious risk both in the United States and other countries. For young people ages fifteen to twenty-four, suicide is the third leading cause of death. In 1997, more teenagers and young adults died from suicide than from cancer, heart disease, AIDS, birth defects, stroke, pneumonia, and influenza combined. For persons between the ages of fifteen and nineteen, firearm-related suicides accounted for 62 percent of the increase in the overall rate of suicide from 1980 through 1997.

Types of Mood Disorders and Diagnostic Criteria

Depression in adults, children, and adolescents has a number of variations. Major depressive disorder is a serious condition characterized by one or more serious episodes. In children and adolescents, this episode lasts an average of seven to nine months and often seems similar to that seen in adults. Typical symptoms include feeling sad, loss of interest or pleasure, considerable self-criticism, and belief that they are inferior to others and are often criticized by others. Such children feel unloved, and they are pessimistic and feel hopeless about the future. They often feel that life is not worth living and they may have thoughts of suicide. However, many times depression in children and adolescents is missed because the symptoms that are seen are behavioral rather than those that seem outwardly to be a depressed mood.

Depressed children and adolescents often are irritable, stubborn, oppositional, and aggressive. Such problems can easily be confused with conduct problems, and depressed children can frequently be misdiagnosed as having conduct or delinquency problems. In addition, very common symptoms of depression in children are poor attention, concentration, and focus. They may be restless and forgetful. Just as is the case with conduct problems, depressed children can be misdiagnosed as suffering from ADHD.

Other symptoms common to children include a lack of energy, trouble sleeping, undereating, or overeating. Different from adults, depressed children often have many more somatic complaints. In fact, they may complain of feeling sick, weak, or unwell, with headaches or stomachaches, and not complain of a depressed mood, again often causing the depression to be overlooked. It is estimated that at any one time, between 10 to 15 percent of children and adolescents have some symptoms of depression. Of those, about 5 percent have major depression (Satcher, 1999a).

Dysthymia

A different type of depression is more chronic. Dysthymic disorder may not have the intensity of symptoms and problems of major depression, but its overall effect upon the child is long term and pervasive. They are depressed most of the time, and these feelings may last for several years. The average length of dysthymia in children is about four years and, as such, children and adults may become so used to their condition that they may no longer complain and even think that this is their usual psychological state. It is not uncommon for both dysthymia and major depression to appear at the same time in the same child. The prevalence of dysthymic disorder in adolescents is estimated to be about 3 percent (Satcher, 1999a). Before puberty, depression is about equally common in boys and girls, but after puberty girls are twice as likely to be depressed.

Bipolar Disorder

Another type of mood disorder, bipolar disorder, is being increasingly understood as a disorder that can be seen in children and adolescents. For many years, it was felt that bipolar disorder did not appear until the late teens or early adulthood. In this older understanding, once termed manic depression, the person would show profound swings of mood. Generally, the first mood seen was depression followed by a period of extreme energy, agitation, and even euphoria, termed mania. In recent years, the understanding of bipolar disorder in children and adolescents has grown considerably. Although it is still typically believed that the first symptoms in bipolar disorder are those of depression, our understanding of how depression in children differs from adults has helped us recognize bipolar disorder at a much earlier age. Now, children who are as young as four or five years of age may be identified as suffering from bipolar disorder. These initial episodes may be the classic depressed mood or may be periods of withdrawal, poor concentration, irritability, oppositional behavior, or aggression. The first manic episodes may not appear for months or even years. As such, the first swings of bipolar disorder in children may be a shift from a normal mood to depression, often without an understandable reason or external stresses.

When mania is seen in children and adolescents, the symptoms are very different from those of depression. Adolescents who experience a manic episode typically feel very energetic, very self-confident, and special or gifted in some way. They tend to have difficulty sleeping but do not get tired. They are often irritable, touchy, and grouchy; at other times, they are seemingly immune to criticism. They may talk a great deal and often very rapidly. They may have many ideas all at the same time and may complain that they feel that their thoughts are racing. They may do their schoolwork far more quickly than usual but in a disorganized, inaccurate way. In extreme states of mania, teenagers may become delusional and grandiose. They may feel that they have special powers or abilities beyond the norm. They may be full of ideas and plans and never carry them out. They may become involved in impulsive, risky, self-defeating behaviors, such as drugs and promiscuity. They may drive cars or motorcycles in a reckless way, and they often become involved in substance abuse. In the most extreme states, they may become very aggressive. Children and adolescents with bipolar disorder are often at substantial risk for suicidal or self-injurious behaviors. In contrast to adults, their mood swings often cycle quite rapidly, even through the course of one day.

Reactive Depression

Probably the most common form of depression in children is reactive depression, or what is often termed *adjustment disorder* with depressed mood. In these cases, the youth experience a depressed mood as a consequence of something happening to them in their environment. Typical events include poor grades, loss of a boyfriend or girlfriend, divorce of parents, academic difficulties, or some sort of failure. In younger children, reactive depression may be sudden and intense and go away fairly rapidly. In adolescents, however, reactive depression may be lengthier and the adolescent may feel lethargic, hopeless, and morose. Sometimes, transient or brief mood swings are seen, but these are not generally thought to be bipolar disorder. One significant problem is the increase of suicides in young children and adolescents as a result of a reactive depression.

Comorbid Disorders

Nearly 65 percent of children and adolescents who are depressed also have other problems, generally called comorbid disorders (Satcher, 1999a). The most common of these are problems with substance abuse, anxiety disorders, or one of the disruptive disorders. Often, the symptoms of depression are seen second, as if a reaction to the other problem, except in the case of substance abuse. It may well be, in fact, that substance abusing young persons are attempting to self-medicate in response to their depression.

Causes of Mood Disorders

Depression and other mood disorders are probably the most researched of all of the emotional and behavioral problems in children and adolescents. Just as there are differing kinds of depression, there are different causes. Today, we believe that there is likely no single cause for depression. Instead, the research points to both biological and environmental or psychosocial causes of depression. As pointed out by the surgeon general (Satcher, 1999a), it is unfortunately the case that most of the research concerning depression has been conducted with adults. To make matters even more complicated, much of the research that has been done with children and adolescents has taken place with people who are already receiving treatment for depression. The possible effect of this is that the research sample is somewhat contaminated or biased. It is, however, what we have to date and with this caution in mind, some very important findings have come to light in recent years.

One intriguing finding is that between 20 and 50 percent of children who have been diagnosed with depression have a family history of depression and that children who have depressed parents are three times more likely to develop depression than are children whose parents are not depressed (Satcher, 1999a). Although these are striking findings, one problem with understanding them is that it is not at all clear how much of this linkage is due to hereditary (genetic) causes and how much is due to the effect upon the family of one or more depressed children. Or, as is even more likely, how do these two causes interact?

When we study the biological symptoms of depression, we see symptoms such as changes in appetite and sleep. These functions are closely related to the functioning of a part of the brain that is deep within the middle brain area or limbic system. In this particular part of the brain, the hypothalamus acts as a regulator for the parts of the body that release specific chemical hormones, or the endocrine system. In particular, the pituitary gland, sometimes called the "master gland," sits at the base of the brain and controls, in part, the release of cortisol and hypo- or hyperthyroidism.

Another very important area of research in depression centers upon what is termed the neuroendocrine system. You may have learned in biology that nerve cells do not really touch one another. Rather, the spark or chemical message jumps a minute gap, the synapse, via chemicals called neurotransmitters. Of particular importance is a subsystem that uses the neurotransmitter serotonin. Many of the most-used antidepressant medications are of a chemical class termed SSRIs, or selective serotonin reuptake inhibitors. Basically, it has been found that in depressed individuals, certain areas of the brain do not efficiently use serotonin. The chemical is released across the synapse. Some, but not enough of it, is absorbed in the receptor areas and bounces back across the synapse to the transmitting brain cell or neuron. The transmitting cell then reabsorbs the unused serotonin. SSRIs block the transmitting cell from reabsorbing the unused serotonin, or the reuptake. This action results in more serotonin being absorbed by the receptor areas of the receiving neuron.

Another very important area of research concerning depression is cognitive or thinking factors. It appears that depressed people have a particular style of thinking. This idea is based upon the concept that often we tend to think, "This happened and I felt that way." But actually it is really, "This happened, I thought about it, and then I felt that way." Depressed individuals tend to have a very pessimistic mind-set. They tend to blame themselves for problems ("My family's problems are all because of me"). They also have a negative view of themselves, the world, and the future ("I am no good, nothing around me is good, and it will only get worse, not better"). We are not certain if these thinking patterns actually cause depression, but we do know that a particular kind of therapy, cognitive-behavioral therapy, acts to change this thinking problem and can be a very effective treatment for some kinds of depression, often in combination with antidepressant medication. Children and teenagers who are depressed often feel hopeless; they see themselves as unworthy, incompetent, and as much less valuable than others. Since children and adolescents often lack the ability to put these thoughts into words, they will act them out behaviorally.

Treatment of Depression

Just as there are many possible causes for depression, so too are there a number of treatment approaches. If a child or teenager acts in the ways described in this chapter, especially if he or she gives indications of thinking about suicide, prompt treatment is essential. The child or adolescent who voices suicidal thoughts, has made a direct threat of suicide, or makes indirect threats should never be left alone until he or she can be seen by a qualified mental health professional. It is, of course, far better to err on the side of caution when one is concerned about a child's welfare.

Counseling or psychotherapy can treat some forms of depression, especially the milder forms alone. Early research on the effectiveness of counseling suggested that various types or schools of thought of counseling were equally effective. Present research does not support this idea. The kind of therapy that works specifically with how the child tends to think, cognitive-behavioral, has been consistently shown to be more effective in the treatment of depression. Because depression affects the family, any counseling with children and teenagers must involve the family. If you are seeking counseling for a depressed young person, it is important to talk with the potential counselor and make certain that the therapist uses cognitive-behavioral therapy and involves the family in treatment.

As the symptoms of depression become more severe, or if counseling alone has not helped, then medication should be considered. For most cases of moderate to severe depression, the combination of cognitive-behavioral therapy, family counseling, and antidepressant medication is likely to be the most helpful. Although pediatricians and family physicians often work with psychotherapists and prescribe antidepressant medication, in cases of severe depression, suicidal thoughts or actions, or bipolar disorder, a child and adolescent psychiatrist must be involved in treatment. The child and adolescent psychiatrist should be a physician who is board certified in child and adolescent psychiatry. Just as it is not appropriate for a counselor who works primarily with adults to treat a child or adolescent, so too must the psychiatrist have specialized training in the assessment and psychiatric treatment of depression. A competent child and adolescent psychiatrist is especially important in the treatment of youth who have comorbid or multiple problems, such as depression and ADHD.

SUICIDE

According to the surgeon general (Satcher, 1999a), in 1996 the age-specific mortality rate from suicide was 1.6 per 100,000 for ten- to fourteen-year-olds, and 9.5 per 100,000 for youth between fifteen and nineteen, which is about six times higher. Younger boys are about four times as likely to commit suicide as girls, and after the late teens girls are twice as likely to commit suicide. Suicide remains a serious problem for our youth and is increasing, especially among minorities. Depressed children are at risk for suicide and both children and adolescents often give out warning signs such as suicidal threats, giving away property, suddenly seeming to feel better, or becoming increasingly withdrawn. In all cases, when a youth makes some sort of suicidal statement or gives some sort of hint, it should be taken very seriously. The child should not be left alone until he or she is carefully evaluated by a mental health professional.

ANGER AND SUBSTANCE ABUSE

One way that anger can be especially problematic is in the development of substance abuse. Although it is believed that some substance abuse problems may well be inherited, we think of them as being risk factors. Thus, having alcoholic parents increases the risk of becoming an alcoholic. Of course, not all children of alcoholics become alcoholics themselves. Some take just the opposite direction and avoid drinking any sort of alcohol. Not all alcoholics have alcoholic parents. Thus, having alcoholic family members is one (although a very strong) risk factor. Other risk factors include anger and depression as well as environmental stress and negative role models. The child who is angry and alienated may turn to alcohol or other drugs because such drugs can initially self-medicate. They can, at first, lessen the emotional discomfort. This initial, temporary reduction in discomfort often results in continued abuse of substances. This continued abuse results in both psychological and physical addiction. Substance abuse can also be reinforced because many substances reduce inhibition. Youth will do or say things when they are intoxicated that they cannot or would not while sober. They can mistakenly begin to believe that substance abuse gives them courage or allows them greater expressive freedom.

A most significant risk for substance abuse is that angry, isolated, and alienated youth often find their way into a negative peer group. In late childhood and adolescence, the peer group holds far more influence than parents or other adult authority figures. This is especially the case when the youth come from dysfunctional and nonsupportive families. Youth such as this are especially vulnerable to negative peer influences. Once engaged with negative peers, they draw themselves further into the peer group and farther from parents and other adults. These youth will support one another and will often provide the emotional connections not found in the home. Thus, the needs that the youth are meeting are perfectly normal. They just can't meet them at home or somewhere else and the negative peer group becomes the primary focus of their lives.

In addition to the self-soothing effect of substance abuse on the angry and alienated child, the psychology of late childhood and adolescent youth is very different from adults. Kids are not little adults. They think in very different ways. One major difference is that young people have a sense of invulnerability. It is not that youth *will* not understand long-term consequences; often they *can't* because their brains have not yet fully developed. A part of the brain, the frontal lobe (especially the left), is responsible for what we call *executive functions*. These executive functions include abstract thinking, impulse control, behavior regulation, and judgment. The frontal lobe grows just as any other part of the body does during childhood. It does not finish growth until mid- to late adolescence. Thus, kids who turn to substances early because of anger and alienation really cannot see the long-term consequences. They may say that they see what substance abuse has done to others, but they really cannot apply it to themselves. They see themselves as being invulnerable and immune to such negative consequences. It is not that they refuse to see the consequences; they simply are not yet developmentally able.

Chapter 6

Anger in Children and Preteens

HOT AND COOL THOUGHTS

In the section on depression, I discussed the thinking or cognitive model as one of the factors in depression. This is much the same in anger. Just as changing how a depressed young person thinks about himself or herself, the world, and the future can reduce or relieve depression, so too can cognitive changes help the angry child. Recall that I suggested it is not so much the question of, "This happened and I felt that way" but instead it is, "This happened, I thought about it, and then I felt that way." The following are some specific examples of how this works.

Jeremiah

Jeremiah always walked to school with a group of friends. He was in the third grade and had had the same set of friends since kindergarten. This year, however, a new child, Bobby, joined the group. Bobby was not really a likeable young man. He was immature, pushy, and self-centered. No one really liked him, but since he lived on their street, he always seemed to join up with the group. One day Bobby was sounding off as usual and no one, as usual, was listening to him. Jeremiah happened to be the unfortunate one who was walking closest to Bobby. Not paying attention at all, Bobby bumped into Jeremiah as he continued his monologue. Jeremiah angrily turned around and shoved Bobby.

In this situation, there are four parts: what happened, what Jeremiah thought about it, what feelings he had after his thoughts, and what he did in response to his feelings. In this case, Bobby bumped into him; Jeremiah thought Bobby did it on purpose (especially since he did not at all care for Bobby). Jeremiah got angry and turned and shoved Bobby. But what if the situation had been different? What if the child talking had not been Bobby but Mikey, one of Jeremiah's friends? What if, since Jeremiah liked Mikey, when Mikey bumped into him, Jeremiah just assumed it to be accidental? Most likely in this situation, Jeremiah would not have gotten angry and most certainly would not have shoved Mikey. Looking at matters this way, we can see that in terms of anger, the process is not really that, "Something happened and I felt that way." Rather, it is "Something happened, I thought about it, and then I felt that way."

The first part of this process of thinking is termed *appraisals.* Appraisals are the way that we characteristically look at things. We tend to look at the same sorts of situations the same way. Once we see it one way, we will likely continue to have that view unless something drastically changes how we look at it. Appraisals result from differing factors. Most of all, they are learned. We encounter a new situation and we don't know what to think about it. We experience and learn from it, and that sets our expectations of similar situations in the future. A very basic example would be how my son developed a fear of gorillas.

Like most parents, we thought that taking four-year-old Josh to the zoo would be a wonderful experience for him. For the most part, this was true, especially the petting zoo. However, all of our good intentions were dashed when we went into the gorilla building. It was an area with two side-entrance ramps that led down to a glassed-in area where the gorillas play. Just as we pushed Josh in his stroller down to the viewing area, a very large gorilla began banging against the glass. Josh was terrified. We quickly left and he seemed to calm down. It looked at first as if we were successful in reassuring him. However, a few nights later, shortly after Josh went to bed, I heard a piercing scream. Running as quickly as I could to his bedroom, I found Josh standing on his bed. In a panic-stricken voice he told me that he had just seen a gorilla in the closet. For the next three or four weeks, before he would settle down for the night, I adopted the ritual of checking his entire room for gorillas. Once reassured that his room was ape free, Josh would be able to go to sleep.

Another part of the cognitive process in anger is not only how we appraise the situation but also how we expect it to turn out. Using an adult example, let's say that your ne'er-do-well brother-in-law is at his usual bar on a Saturday night. Someone bumps into him. He decides that the person bumped into him on purpose. He becomes angry. In the past, he has been in a number of fistfights and has most often come out the winner. So, he wheels around, cocks his fist and sees

Mike Tyson, the heavyweight boxer. Odds are that his expectations of the success of his past fighting behavior will change. If he has any sense at all, he will turn his other shoulder to him and say, "Excuse me, Mr. Tyson, sir. Would you like to bump into my other arm?" But what if he gets bumped, decides that it was done on purpose, and turns around to find another Michael—Michael Jackson? Most likely your brother-in-law's expectations would be different between the two Michaels. (Unless of course your brother-in-law is still the same lunatic he has always been.)

With children, we can talk about it in terms of "hot thoughts" and "cool thoughts." Hot thoughts, of course, are those thoughts that automatically make us angry. In the case of Jeremiah and Bobby, it was—"He did it on purpose, just like he always does." A cool thought, of course, would be that it was an accident. We can teach our children to think of situations in differing ways. A hot thought can be replaced with a cool thought. In this example, even if Jeremiah believed that Bobby did it on purpose, a cool thought could be, "It's just not worth it."

If your child is one who tends to automatically appraise situations in a way that makes him or her angry, then practicing cool thoughts can be a very good way to help him or her learn to manage anger. One way that I like to use is to keep a little logbook. At the end of the school day, sit down with your child and ask him or her to come up with one or two things that gave rise to the feeling of anger. Ask what he or she was thinking at the time. See if your child can come up with a cool thought instead. It helps sometimes to keep a piece of paper with one side titled Hot Thoughts and the other titled Cool Thoughts. Make it a game. See how many different cool thoughts your child can produce. After some practice in coming up with cool thoughts, ask him or her to tell you of a situation in which he or she could have had a hot thought and instead replaced it with a cool thought. Some parents like to give little rewards or prizes for such times and some children respond very well to that.

Although this can work very well, one of the potential problems that parents of angry children can experience is that their children are not really talkers or philosophers. They are action oriented. This is especially the case with children who have problems with aggression. Children and teenagers who are aggressive tend to have a fairly concrete or nonimaginative way of looking at things. They are especially prone to looking at the same situation in the same way over and over again, regardless of the success of that particular viewpoint. To make matters even more difficult, they are not particularity verbal persons. When you ask them to think about how they think, all you get, if you are lucky, is a puzzled look and maybe a grunt. That is because we have learned that youth with anger problems tend to be very concrete in how they look at situations. They don't have the skill of cognitive flexibility: the skill to be able to understand that a situation can be interpreted in a number of different ways.

This is especially true with younger children who are very egocentric by nature in their worldview. Because of where they are in their growth and development they simply cannot imagine that anyone would see things differently from their view. The problem is, of course, that talking to a nonverbal child about looking at situations differently holds very little promise of success. Instead, parents can try a game each night to teach the skills of cognitive flexibility. Take some cartoons and block or cut out the captions or balloons that hold the captions. Make a game of coming up with as many differing things that the cartoon character is saying. Have as much fun as possible and think of the wildest things to say. As the child enjoys the game, he or she is also learning how to look at situations in a different way.

Sometimes, if your child is not much of a talker at all, you can use other ways or "paths" to communicate. Rather than asking your child to relate experiences, have him or her draw what happened. You can even draw alternative ways of looking at things in response to your child's drawing. Again, have as much fun as possible doing this activity. If your child isn't much of an artist or feels inhibited about drawing, then cut pictures from the newspaper or magazines and make a collage that tells the story. Often, when I work with a child who has been a "counseling failure" in learning anger management, I have found that the child simply is not a verbal person. Using art as a means of communication has opened up all sorts of avenues for these previously untreatable children.

FEELINGS

Just as we can change how a child looks at a situation, we can also change how that child responds emotionally to a situation. Children with anger-management problems often have a very limited range of emotions. They are happy, mad, sad, or glad. They don't know the difference between being angry and irritated. For them, there are no shades of gray. It is either black or white. Children with anger problems typically do not have subtle emotions. Beyond that, they often move from a nonangry state to an angry state in the blink of an eye. Research with persons who have anger-management problems has shown that some individuals move more quickly to an angry state and sometimes, when they reach that state, are unable to either calm themselves down or be calmed down by others. For some, this problem is so severe that they are seen as having an actual mental disorder.

Intermittent Explosive Disorder

The diagnosis of intermittent explosive disorder is given to children and adults who, for the most part, hold their temper in and then suddenly reach a point where they explode in anger. Often this happens to the great surprise of the person as well as those around him or her. When these people reach a certain point of anger, there is simply no turning around. No reasoning will calm them and no consequence will deter them. Although every child has temper tantrums, children with intermittent explosive disorder go far beyond the normal response to frustration that is a temper tantrum. Adults, of course, can lose their tempers and can act in ways that are completely out of character. Add the mix of alcohol or other drugs or some underlying serious emotional disturbance and the possibility for explosive behavior increases.

In some individuals, there seems to be no clear underlying cause and the loss of temper is chronic and destructive. In the DSM-IV the diagnostic criteria for intermittent explosive disorder are as follows:

A. Several discrete episodes of failure to resist aggressive impulses that result in serious assaultive acts or destruction of property.
B. The degree of aggressiveness expressed during the episode is grossly out of proportion to any precipitating psychosocial stressors.
C. The aggressive episodes are not better accounted for by another mental disorder and are not due to the direct physiological effects of a substance or a general medical condition (p. 612). (Re-

printed with permission from the *Diagnostic and Statistical Manual of Mental Disorders,* Fourth Edition. Copyright 1994, American Psychiatric Association.)

The cause of intermittent explosive disorder is unknown and it was once thought to be a relatively rare condition. It is thought, however, in recent studies, that intermittent explosive disorder may be an underdiagnosed condition and that persons who suffer from it are now thought of as having character problems. Studies of the brain using neural imaging do suggest that there are differences deep in the brain structures of persons with intermittent explosive disorder, especially in the limbic system. Other neurological studies have shown problems in the functioning of the prefrontal cortex of the brain. Some suggest that an imbalance in the neurotransmitter serotonin may be responsible for the outbursts. Other factors that have been linked to intermittent explosive disorder include a history of being victimized by violence or abuse or exposure to violence.

There is no cutoff line between a normal temper and intermittent explosive disorder. It is best viewed as a continuum. On one end of the line, we have the children who sometimes have outbursts of anger. The children who meet the DSM-IV criteria for intermittent explosive disorder would be on the other end of that imaginary line. Most children with temper problems fall somewhere in the middle. They have temper problems beyond that of most children their age but not so much that they meet diagnostic criteria. These children are different in how they experience and express anger. Often, anger just seems to come over them. Later, after the eruption, someone can ask the children what came over them and they will honestly answer that they have no idea. They seem to move very quickly to the angry side.

Part of this rapid movement comes from what we talked about earlier in the way that a chronically angry person habitually looks at a situation in a manner that makes the anger response more likely. Another part of this rapid movement may result from being exposed to role models such as parents or media that promote a rapid escalation to violence and aggression. Other reasons, as is the case with intermittent explosive disorder, may be biological. Children with ADHD, especially those of the hyperactive-impulsive type, can have very quick tempers. Children who are moody due to an imbalance of serotonin can also be easily angered. In fact, in young children, irritability and anger problems are often a more common symptom of depression than a sad mood or crying.

Some children move to quick anger with almost any irritant. But these are the uncommon ones. Most children have certain "hot buttons" or issues that trigger an angry emotional response. In these specific situations, children move much more quickly to an angry state. Very young children, because they have both a limited range of developed emotions and because they tend to be very egocentric, often become quickly angry over situations such as wanting another child's cookie or shoving a child in order to grab a toy.

School-age children have developed a wider range of emotions. Emotions mature and become more complex in much the same manner as thinking abilities mature. In school-age children, verbal skills are learned and often used in anger. They have a great range of options than simply physical aggression. Young girls, who tend to develop verbally before young boys, often show more verbal and social aggression at these ages. Of course, this verbal aggression can be just as painful and significant as physical aggression, for both boys and girls. But because verbal aggression is not as easily seen by adults or perhaps even appreciated, this kind of aggression is wrongly thought of as being different and even less consequential than physical aggression. Typically, aggression in school-age children, either physical or verbal, is directed at someone else rather than a simple temper tantrum or outburst as a result of frustration. School-age children can show their anger by destroying the property of someone else, by bullying, and by verbal attacks. Because the school-age child is still growing psychologically, he or she often has the very difficult problem of being able to feel new emotions but not yet having the verbal or physical tools to express that anger. Thus, even though a child may be able to understand more complicated emotions, the abilities for communicating these feelings have not yet caught up with the emotional development. As a result, he or she may have many emotions but only a few ways, including aggression, to express them.

Preteenagers continue in this complex struggle between feeling many more new emotions and not yet having the resources to express them. Although the adolescents may be able to feel more complex emotions, they have not yet caught up in their ability to think and reason abstractly. For example, it seems that preteenagers are perpetually concerned about fairness. A preteenager may feel unfairly treated in a certain situation. They know the feeling but cannot yet put words to, or explain, why they believe they are being treated unfairly or differently. This is the origin of that timeless phrase, "But Mom, all the other kids get to . . . ." I am virtually certain that even in ancient Rome, the mantra "But Dad, all the other kids get to go to the coliseum" was heard far more than the words of Virgil or the speeches of Caesar. With preteenagers, the "hot buttons" tend to be such things as arguing about limits on time and actions, association with other peers, and expecting privileges in spite of poor performance on required chores or tasks.

COOLING DOWN

In the case of the child or adolescent who truly gets to a point where his or her anger is explosive, the critical thing to do is to avoid getting there. Once the child has reached that point, not much productive can be done. When he or she is at that stage of rage, no reasoning is possible. It is not a matter of the child who *won't* calm his or her anger, but rather when he or she gets to this point the child simply *can't*. Thus, when a child reaches a certain level of anger, it is pointless to try to argue, persuade, or debate a point. The physical potential of the anger needs to be contained and the discussion deferred to a later moment. Parents of children who have explosive anger typically learn the "hot buttons" of their children and can often see the physical response of anger even before their children can.

In research of angry persons, it has been found that children and adults with chronic anger problems have much more difficulty responding to "proprioceptive" stimuli. Translated, this means that people with chronic anger problems don't "listen to their bodies" as well as others do. Generally, when we experience an emotion, we feel it somewhere in our body. Often, in times of stress, we can feel our shoulders tighten, we feel the blood rush to our faces, and we experience our hearts beating faster. But persons with chronic anger problems have much more difficulty doing that. They misread, or don't read at all, the signals sent to them by their bodies. They can even be red-faced, huffing and puffing, oblivious to the whole world but not to themselves. For such children, when they are asked what came over them, the answer "I don't know" is genuine and truthful.

Response to this problem really exists on two levels. The first is at a prevention level. Children can be taught to recognize the hot buttons. Once they have done that, then, in peaceful moments, parents and child can develop an anger plan that allows the child to have constructive way of expressing anger. For example, if a hot button is going to bed, the plan might be, "I get mad when Mommy and Daddy tell me to go to bed. When I get mad, I throw things and get into trouble. Next time I get mad at having to go to bed, I will take three deep breaths. If I am able to not throw things because I took three breathes for two days in a row, I will get a reward." But what about the child who cannot even feel when the button is being pushed? Parents in these situations should work with how the child feels his or her body in areas other than anger. When taking the child for a walk, they can talk with the child about how the grass under his or her feet feels different from the concrete sidewalk. When the child listens to music that has a certain emotion, the parent can ask the child what feeling that song brings. Or, in another way, the parent can use colors and ask the child what feeling goes with what color. The point to all of this is practice. The better able the child is to identify hot buttons and feelings early on, the better able the child and parent are at avoiding an angry confrontation.

Not all things are worth fighting about. Parents should take some time before an anger episode and list the issues that are hot buttons. Then, the parents should think of three containers or cases to put those issues in. There is the basket that simply is not negotiable. For example, homework must be done, or children should not play with matches. Then, there is a second case that is negotiable. For example, even though homework must be done, the time that the homework is done often can be open for negotiation. The point, after all, is to get the homework done, not get caught in long power struggles over when that work is to be accomplished. Kids can learn pretty quickly that if they simply argue and argue, enough time is wasted that they can avoid the homework. So, instead, without opportunity for discussion, in a calm manner, simply say to the child that the homework needs to be done by such and such a time. If not, a specific consequence will follow and there is no room for discussion. Third, there are the cases that really aren't all that important anyway. One such case might be that of hairstyle. Another might be that of certain clothing or other apparel. Look back in your own life and think about those things that seemed so important to you when you were a child that aren't so crucial now. If you do this, you can quickly add to the case of topics not really worth getting all that excited about.

ANGER PLANS

Some years back, there was a catch phrase, "teachable moments." The idea was that at certain times things happen that can be learning experiences. For example, when an adult notices a child really trying hard at something but simply missing the mark, the adult can step in and use the motivation of the child at that moment to teach a skill. Other times, the phrase refers to just after an event or behavior when the adult can sit down and process with the child what had just gone on in a way that the child can learn from the experience. For most kids, anger episodes are not teachable moments. The youth is too emotionally aroused to take the needed intellectual steps back to look at what happened and why. Often, the adult is much the same way. It is hard to teach when puffs of steam are coming out of your ears, after all. And, of course, often in conflicts between parents and children, there are winners and there are losers. It would be wonderful if the old "win-win" concept really worked most of the time with kids, but it doesn't. They must set limits. Parents must set and enforce rules and consequences. It is fairly rare for a youth sitting in time-out to think of his situation as a "win-win."

What is a parent to do? One distinct advantage that we have as adults is the ability to plan and think in perspective. As adults, we are much better prepared to think in advance about situations in which children can become angry. We can also think about specific strategies to assist them in learning to manage their anger. In other words, we can prepare an anger plan. An anger plan is simply thinking about which situations could trigger anger and coming up with strategies to teach children how to manage that anger and to negotiate the stressful situation when anger is felt.

For example, a common area of conflict is bedtime. As children grow older, they want to stay up later. The reasons are natural. As they grow, they want to feel more in charge of their lives. They develop a stronger sense of identity and consequently want to test limits. Their range of interest expands and sometimes the things that interest them, such as television shows, are on past their bedtime. Or, if they have older siblings, they want to be like them, including the time to go to bed.

When a child has an 8:30 p.m. bedtime, 8:35 is not a teachable moment. The stakes are too high and the emotions too charged. Instead, the parent should pick a time when the child is in a good mood, not tired, and not a few moments away from going to bed. The parent can initiate the talk by saying that going to bed on time is good way to earn points, stars, later bedtimes on nonschool nights, or whatever reward system is being used to encourage positive behavior. The parent can also remind the child that there are consequences if bedtime is not followed and that neither the parent nor the child really wants those consequences to happen. The parent then can say that he or she knows that kids really do think bedtime is important and that there are fun things that a child naturally wants to do.

Kids know that sleep is needed, even though they may not want to acknowledge it. So, the parent could suggest to the child that rather than waiting for the problem to happen, they should sit down and make a bedtime plan that includes what to do if the child feels really angry and frustrated about having to go to bed. Ask the child for some suggestions about how to release anger and have some of your own available to use as illustrations. For example, a child angry about having to go to bed might need a way to express that anger through a drawing or making an allowable and appropriate verbal or nonverbal expression of that anger. Anger plans don't stop at the moment of anger. If the youth does manage his or her anger, then that should be noticed and praised. If the child does not, then later on, perhaps the next day, when cooler heads prevail, the incident should be discussed in a nonpunitive way. Successful anger plans often follow the model used in Box 6.1.

The anger plan involves a series of parts. First, prior to the event, the circumstances are discussed. Second, the plan is written. Or, in the case of younger children or youth who learn better by seeing rather than hearing, the plan is portrayed using drawings or photographs. The plan is then posted somewhere visible when the critical situation does happen. After all, in the heat of anger, things are forgotten. The use of a posted plan can sometimes provide helpful reminders of both anger cues and ways to manage the anger. The last component, practice, is the one most often left out and can be the most important part of the plan. Children learn by doing. Simply put,

---

Box 6.1. Anger Plan Model

1. Identify the possible situation in advance.
2. Understand the feelings and reasons behind the anger.
3. Plan in advance how to express feelings in an appropriate way.
4. Identify cues or signals that the adult can give to the child to clue him or her in on the need to use the plan.
5. Identify the self-talk (e.g., hot or cool thoughts) that directs behavior.
6. Write out the plan; use drawings or photographs if needed.
7. Post the plan where it can be easily seen in a moment of anger.
8. Follow through on the plan.
9. Reward and praise for compliance.
10. Follow through on consequences if the plan is not followed.
11. Have a "chalk talk" and discuss what happened later, when emotions have cooled.
12. Practice using the plan before the situation arises.

---

kids need repetition and practice until they get it right. But as any parent who has tried to have a child learn music well knows, practice is boring, especially when a person is practicing something not all that important or interesting. For this reason, parents should try to make a game of practicing anger-management skills and rewarding in the practice session when the child follows through with appropriate behaviors. Some families have gone to the practice of "mad drills" as a way to promote what to do in "emotional emergencies." Others have used camcorders to produce fun videos about what to do that can be watched again. Certain creative families have even developed an "Anger Academy Award" ceremony to congratulate the youth on his or her production.

Anger plans aren't permanent. What works for a while will not always work for an extended period of time. Part of the anger plan has to be a time for review and modification. Children quickly tire of specific rewards, especially if they have ADHD or some other problem with impulsiveness. Parents then become frustrated and give up on the plan. The problem is not the plan. It did work. The problem is that the reward became boring. To address this, parents should, at the time of putting together the anger plan, say to the child that the rewards that seem good now will lose their value later on as he or she gets used to them. At that point, parents can sit down and come up with a list of possible rewards that can be used when the child tires of the one currently used. In addition, explain to the child that it is important to monitor the plan and make sure that it is still working. One way, of course, to do that is to look at the results: Does the child go to bed? Does the child earn his or her rewards? Another way, one that provides for greater opportunity to teach and learn, is to plan a regular time to sit down and talk over how things are going. Debriefing sessions are critical parts of any anger plan. But the debriefing should not be reserved for only those times after something happens (or doesn't happen). Rather, the parents should schedule regular times to sit down as a family and talk about how well the plans are working and make the needed changes to assure continued success of the plan.

Sometimes, parents object to using reward systems. They feel that they are bribing their kids or teaching them to expect something for what is really required behavior. If you think about it, we all work on a reward system. We go to work and are paid for our efforts. In a sense, learning how to behave appropriately and to manage anger is an important part of the "job" of being a child. Looking at things this way can often make using reward plans far more appealing to parents. This is not to advocate that children should be turned into little businesspersons who expect some sort of gain for every action. The most effective reward for children continues to be the attention and approval of significant adults in their lives. When a reward is given, it should always be paired with sincere praise and statements of approval. Later, as the children gain better behavioral control, the use of specific rewards can be "faded" or reduced away until the only reward is the approval of the parents. However, that will not always be enough, and parents should be ready to return to a structured reward system early on if problems reappear.

Kids often have more than one or two significant adults in their lives, and parents can draw upon this to build a network of praise. They can involve grandparents, older siblings, teachers, or any other significant older person in the plan. Such persons can be made aware of the plan and rewards so that they can also offer rewards and praise when circumstances are appropriate. Even if these other persons don't have the opportunity to directly implement the plan (such as grandparents who live a long distance away), parents can tell them of the plan and the adults can bring up the successes in a conversation and provide the children with additional sources of adult recognition and approval.

WHAT IF ALL THIS STUFF FAILS?

I think the problem with most books about dealing with angry children is that the impression is given that all of these ideas seem to just work magically. All a parent needs to do is to read the book, make a couple of changes, and there he or she has it, a perfect child. If only it were so and if only kids never lost their temper in the grocery store. So, what to do when things go wrong?

Time-Out

The most effective consequence known in research with changing behavior in children is time-out. Time-out is not a punishment. It is a specific technique that results in behavior change. The first thing you need to know about time-out is that you should never use it unless you plan to follow through with it. Never make empty threats with time-out. Kids will quickly learn that you don't mean business. Don't use time-out as a surprise. Instead, plan ahead. Tell the child in advance what behaviors are expected and what consequences, such as time-out, will follow. You can discuss time-out when you put together your anger plan. When you do use time-out, always praise the child if he or she follows the command on the first prompt, but don't expect miracles. I do recall one child who, after he lost his temper, composed himself, saw what he did, and marched over and sat in the time-out chair. When the children do comply, make certain that you praise them.

Some specific suggestions have been adapted from Russell Barkley's (1997) excellent resource for clinicians who work with defiant children. First of all, when parents tell a child to go into time-out, it needs to be a command, not a request. We are not talking about a drill sergeant here. You should not yell at your child. Instead, use a firm, clear, direct, and businesslike tone. Tell the child in very specific terms what you want. For example, "Jimmy, turn off the television now."

Of course, when he hears you, Jimmy will jump right up, turn off the television, pausing only to ask you if you want him to do the dishes on the way. Not surprisingly, most kids don't want to turn off the television and most certainly don't rush to do so. To manage this, parents should count backward from either seven or five, out loud, one second at a time. Later on, parents don't need to do the countdown but simply tell the child that he or she has a certain number of seconds to comply. Immediately upon hearing this, your child will recognize the error of his or her ways and skip happily to act on your request. More likely, you will need to make direct eye contact with the child, raise your voice up one notch, stand in a firm manner, and say, "Jimmy, if you don't turn off the televison, you will have to sit in the time-out chair." Once you give this warning, it is time for mission control again, counting backward. If the child still refuses to go, immediately go over, pick him or her up, and put the child in time-out. If he or she resists, use slight physical force, but never so much as to risk injury. Once in the chair, the child is to stay there for the mandated time. There are to be no bathroom breaks or further arguments. Say to the child in a firm voice, "You will stay here until I tell you to get up." Then, say no more. If you need to, say only that you are not coming back to the chair until he or she is quiet. Never argue with the child when he or she is in time-out. When the appropriate time is up, return to the child. Repeat the command. If he or she complies, give praise. If he or she does not comply, then tell him or her that it is time for another round in the chair. Give the child one warning and walk away if there is no compliance.

Time-out is an art form, and as such, has certain qualities. Time-out is absolute. If the child leaves the time-out chair, there must be a consequence. Again, in the anger-management plan, the cost of leaving the time-out chair is spelled out in advance. Such consequences can be the loss of television time, early bedtime, loss of points or stars in a behavioral system, or loss of other privileges such as the use of a favorite toy for a certain period of time. If you have a child who tends to not follow the time-out rules, then further advance planning is needed. Take all of the toys, radios, video games, televisions, and other major play items from the child's room. When the child refuses to go to time-out, he or she is given one warning, one countdown, and then taken to the bedroom and told to sit on the edge of the bed for the specified time. Keep the door open, but if the child leaves, then immediately assign another consequence. Either in the time-out chair or on the bed, there is only one way to sit. That way is with both buttock cheeks firmly on the seat or bed. The chair should be straight-backed and uncomfortable. The chair should not face anything of interest and usually is placed in a corner—far enough away from the wall so that the child can't kick it. Never use bathrooms, closets, or the child's bedroom for chair placement. Instead, place it in an area that can be observed as the adults continue on with their business. When the child does comply and is ready to leave, make certain to praise him or her. Try not to start with going to bed as the first problem to be addressed with time-out. Pick out another problem and get to the point where time-out begins to work before attempting to use it as a means to get the child to go to bed.

Time-out has its own laws about time. The general rule of thumb is one to two minutes per year. Thus, for a five-year-old, time-out should be ten to twenty minutes. Typically, I have found that time-out never works quickly. It fails generally because the kids outlast the parents. I am not at all surprised when the first episodes of time-out go for at least thirty minutes up to two hours before the child quiets down. It may take several weeks before time-out really works. Parents need to steel themselves to outlast their children. Remember, in the end, you are teaching your child self-discipline and control. Without these qualities, trouble will surely follow when your child gets older.

Problems are also frequently encountered in public places. Angry children don't just have outbursts at home and parents need to be prepared to manage situations in places such as stores and automobiles. Since it is not really very practical to always strap the time-out chair on your (or your child's) back whenever you go out, planning is essential. Before you go anywhere, make certain that you lay out the rules for behavior in advance and the rewards and consequences that will follow. Make certain that you are clear what the rewards will be if the child follows the rules and the specific consequences if the rules are not followed. When you get to your destination, before you leave the car, go over the rules and results. If the child refuses, have a time-out in the car.

Although some adults have trouble believing it, not all the things we do are engrossing and fascinating to children. Grocery shopping and Laundromats are just two specific examples. In such cases the prudent parent brings along an activity or two to keep the child busy.

Don't feel that every activity has to have a social or educational value. Remember, in such situations, your objective is to keep the child busy, not teach him or her piano.

There are some very specific places and circumstances in which kids seem to love to act out. One of those is in the store. Many children seem to thrive on an audience and do whatever they can to get one when they decide to misbehave. If you are familiar with the store, pick out a place that is generally pretty empty as the place you will go for time-out. If you don't know the store, then think of using places such as changing rooms or men's suits. Grocery stores are pretty difficult to find quiet places. Sometimes, you may have to employ other consequences, such as loss of a privilege after the store, for example, no television time. When dining out, rest rooms are a good option, as are car time-outs or loss of privileges later on.

When all else fails, you still have options. Carry a notebook and when the child begins to act out tell him or her that if you have to put a checkmark down, then there will be a later consequence. In good weather, you can take the child outside and have him or her face a wall, but be certain there is no danger of the child running away and into traffic. The same goes for use of the car as a time-out place. Most often, the best alternative is the notebook.

Chapter 7

Anger in Teenagers

More years back than I care to state, I was in training under a well-known adolescent forensic psychiatrist. Like most interns, I would seek a moment when I could ask a "penetrating" question. (My motivation of course was not so much to seek an answer but to impress him with the depth of my thinking.) After a difficult interview with a particularly obstinate young offender, I asked my clinical supervisor just what he thought was the true answer to preventing juvenile delinquency. Allocating as much thought as such an inane question deserved, he paused briefly and said that the only real answer was to build a fence around a state (we can pick on Indiana, I suppose) and mandate that all persons between the ages of twelve and eighteen be kept there. They would be released only when they reached the age of majority and were, therefore, legally adults and legally responsible. Since there would be no juveniles, there could be no juvenile delinquency. I didn't know whether to laugh, change the subject, or simply crawl away.

As adolescents will gladly (and most likely repeatedly) tell you, they are no longer children. What works for children will not work for teenagers. For example, time-out and point systems are ineffective after a certain age. Teenagers are not really suitable for time-out (unless of course you have an uncle and aunt with a fenced-in farm in Indiana). Time-out or point systems tend to lose effectiveness between the ages of twelve and thirteen. Some youth who are socially immature may still respond to such systems, but they are rare.

Teenagers are not yet adults and are no longer children for a number of reasons. Of course, societal pressures and expectations change as youth grow older. Adolescents are given more responsibility and are expected to be more responsible. The demands in school increase as does the complexity of the work. Teenagers begin to think about careers and vocations. Socially, they become more focused upon their peer group than upon the family and psychologically move toward more independence as they begin to develop their own sense of personal identity. They are more sensitive to what others, especially their peers, think of them. They confront substantial life decisions such as substance abuse, sexuality, and the choice of friends.

Their bodies change, too. Not only do changes result from hormones surging through them, but their brains also change. The frontal lobe, the area responsible for planning, judgment, abstract thinking, and other more complex or executive functions, begins to develop in both area and complexity. These changes mean that teenagers think and feel in ways very different from both children and adults. They are more complex and well developed cognitively and emotionally than children, but are not yet adults.

Adolescents are unique. They are neither old children nor young adults. They are young persons who are going through the healthy, normal developmental processes of becoming more independent, of developing a sense of personal identity that is separate and distinct from their parents and siblings, and of preparing themselves for eventually separating from the family and living on their own as young adults. Although such times can be trying and difficult even in the best of families, one important thing to keep in mind is that the stereotype that adolescents are all troubled and conflicted simply because they are teenagers is a myth. Developmental research concerning adolescents consistently demonstrates that, as a whole, teenagers are emotionally healthy and behaviorally stable. They are better than we think. Some youth certainly do have serious problems, but most do not. Often, what is at the bottom of conflict between teenagers and parents is the healthy tension between the adolescents' desires to become more independent and the parents' natural protectiveness about their youth. Teenagers do not have the ability yet to think through consequences. Since their life experiences are much fewer, they don't have the perspective that adults have. But since they so strongly desire to be their own person, accepting the limits placed upon them by parents can be very difficult.

Generally, it is not so much what the limit is, but how the parent puts that limit into place and how that limit is applied. In order to be able to effectively place limits on negative behaviors, it is essential that parents consistently be on the lookout for and praise good behavior. In more than thirty years of practice with adolescents, I have yet to see even one youth who is negative all of the time. Granted, the average teenager's behavior can be disruptive, often at the most inconvenient times. I think that adolescents have a collective understanding that the time to not "have anything to wear" is directly related to the pressing need of the parents to get someplace. Without fail, the moment a parent is running late is the exact moment when the teenager discovers he or she has simply no clothes that could conceivably be worn in public. This is especially the case with teenagers who have ADHD or other disruptive behavior disorders. Their greatest struggle is planning ahead. Time crunches, therefore, are by definition minefields for conflict. But, even with the most exasperatingly procrastinating teen, there is bound to be at least one time when the youth is actually ready when the parent needs to go. In those moments (just before you pass out from the shock) make certain to praise the young person for being ready.

I often ask parents to list the annoying behaviors of their teenagers and what they have done about it. The list of problems grows quickly, as does the list of unsuccessful interventions to change the behavior. Then, when the question is asked in the other direction, "What did your teenager do right and how did you reward it?" the list becomes much shorter. Often, parents, to their chagrin, acknowledge that they are so relieved that no conflict or misbehavior occurred that they forget to acknowledge or reward the youth. Other times, parents may simply take for granted the many times that the youth does comply and is not disruptive or difficult.

For this reason, when I meet with parents for the first time, after I take in the litany of problems, I ask them to spend the next week looking in the opposite direction and come back to me with a list, no matter how short, of what the youth did right. If in the first session they are able to make such a list, we can go ahead to the next step that is often reserved for the second meeting, which is to find just one or two minor problems that appear every now and then and target them by making certain that he or she is praised when he or she doesn't do the negative behavior that the parent usually expects. Thus, when the youth is actually on time for breakfast, or does get homework done on time, or even simply waits his or her turn, the parent uses that moment to praise and acknowledge the positive behavior, no matter how seemingly minor or inconsequential.

To illustrate, a parent may, at the table, ask the youth to pass the bread. When the youth does so, the parent can then take the opportunity to stop, thank the youth for passing the bread, and state how much he or she appreciates it when the young person responds in a positive manner to a request. In this case, it is not so much what the youth has done, but the fact that the youth has done something and is receiving praise. The critical piece to this is not so much that you can begin to feel confident in your ability to get your teen to pass you bread but rather that you have taken control.

Parents often feel that they have no control over their teens, when in actuality, they have a great deal of control. When we typically think of control and adolescents, we most often turn to the big things: staying out late at night, choice of friends, choice of music, and so on. In so doing, we neglect the smaller, even more important parts of their lives that we do control. Ultimately, we really have no control over how another person acts. What we do have control over is how we respond to that person. One never sees dramatic changes in a teenager's behavior. Instead, one sees small steps that, when taken together, look dramatic. Parents can and should control how they respond in a positive manner to their youth's positive behavior. Without this first step, managing the more negative and disruptive behaviors in an effective way will never happen.

For this reason, it is important that parents of teenagers spend positive one-on-one time with their youth. The time needn't be either long or forced. It is essential to do two things during that time. First, find something that the youth is doing that is deserving of praise and acknowledge it in a meaningful and not overly showy way. Second, because your kid is a kid, after all, he or she will likely do some kind of minor misbehavior or slightly obnoxious behavior during the time that you are with him or her. Ignore it. Don't waste your energy and squander the opportunity for positive time on something that, in the long run, really means little.

Beyond the essential need to attend to and reward positive behavior, effective discipline with adolescents has some very specific components. First of all, parents need to be clear and unambiguous. One of my favorite examples revolves around the eternal homework question. Generally, parents want their kids to do homework and kids don't want to. Homework is not fun. It is work. I doubt seriously that changing the term to "homefun" would make much difference (other than to fully convince your teenager that you have totally fallen off of the deep end). What teenager really wants and likes to do homework? I often tell parents, in front of their kids who nod enthusiastically, that I am more worried about the kid who likes to do homework than the kid who abhors it and does everything that he or she can to avoid doing it. When parents reflect back to their own attitude about homework and how much they preferred spending time with their friends or watching television to spending a rewarding hour with an algebra book, if honest, they would quickly acknowledge that homework is a pain. But homework must be done, painful as it is, boring as it is.

Adults must go to work. They have their jobs and kids have theirs. Problem is, adults have some choice about the kind of job they do or can see some type of immediate reward (e.g., a paycheck) for working. With kids and homework, the benefits are much less obvious and clear. Generally, the benefit of doing your homework is that you get a good grade and your parents don't punish you. The typical teenager, in faultless logic, can reason in one of two ways: They do not like to get grief from their parents. So, they can do the homework and avoid the grief. Or the industrious teenager can attempt to figure out a way to wear his or her parents down so they no longer give grief when the homework doesn't get done. This, of course, is the perfect solution: no homework and no grief. If only that could be so! Looking at it from this perspective, is it any wonder that getting your adolescents to do homework is a struggle?

For that reason, I suggest that when the time comes to tell the youth to do homework, do not ask the question, "Would you like to do your homework now?" The answer is evident: of course not. But, there is more than the obvious going on here. Asking the question, "Would you like to do your homework?" is ambiguous because it gives the youth an out. When given the choice, he or she will avoid doing something disagreeable. So, instead of giving commands with a question, give commands in clear and specific ways. The correct phrase is, "It is time to do your homework." There needs to be no discussion, no negotiating, and no gratitude when it is finally done. When your youth are doing their homework, they are not doing you a favor. They are doing what they are supposed to do. So, there is no need for a parent to thank a youth for doing what that youth is supposed to do.

There is a need to give a clear and specific expectation with clear directions and follow through. The follow through as a result of completing homework needs to be some type of privilege or reward if work is done or a consequence or loss of privilege if it is not done— no dramatics, nothing more than what we as adults expect out of our own lives. If we go to work, we get paid. If we don't, we lose our jobs and starve. The end.

It is at this point that those readers who have children not yet old enough to be teenagers will pause and say to themselves, "Wow, how logical that is. I know that I am having trouble with my child now, but I can't wait until he or she grows into a teenager. Sounds like it will be much more logical and a lot easier then!" Simultaneously, those readers who do have teenagers may spout appropriate foul language toward any dimwitted psychologist who would think that such a simplistic solution would work for their kids.

ADOLESCENTS AND BEHAVIOR MANAGEMENT

In order to think this through, we need to turn back to research on the effective principles for managing the behavior of teenagers. Just as with younger children, discipline is not punishment or negative consequences alone. Discipline is a method of teaching. Disciplining a youth is a combination of both rewarding the good behavior and providing negative consequences for the undesired behavior. Punishing youth without teaching them or giving them the opportunity to learn an alternative behavior is not only ineffective, but dooms the youth to repeat the same problem behaviors over and over again. When you give a youth only a negative consequence without first offering positive consequences for desired behavior, a cycle of negativity begins that typically only ends in anger, frustration, and increased negative behavior. Thus, parents should never punish a youth unless that youth has first had the opportunity to earn some sort of reward for doing the right thing.

Typically, when I see a family, the parents have become so frustrated by the problematic behavior of the youth that all they focus on are negative consequences. By the time I see them, they have taken away nearly all of the positives in that youth's life. The youth is grounded until the next century; the television, radio, video games, computer, telephone, telegraph, and carrier pigeons have all been taken away. The kid, seeing no end to it all, figures he or she has nothing to lose, so why even bother changing? I tell the parents to give half of the privileges back that very moment and to set up a system in which the other half can be earned through positive behavior. Then, hopefully, if the youth has something to gain and something to lose, we have a toehold on turning things around. More simply put in the words of my grandmother, "You catch more flies with honey than you do with vinegar."

Before implementing any kind of system of negative consequences, parents need to first very specifically state what it is they want from their youth. The desired behavior needs to be clear, focused, and specific, such as, "You will have your homework done by nine o'clock." Next, the positive consequence needs also to be clearly put forth: "When you get your homework done, you can watch an hour of television. If you get all of your homework done on each school night by nine o'clock, you can stay up an extra hour on weekends." Critical here is the specificity of the desired behavior and the specificity of the reward. Nothing is unclear or ambiguous. It does no good to offer such a system if the youth doesn't know how to accomplish the goals. Often as parents, we assume that youth know how to do something— even something as simple as organizing homework. Before you implement a reward plan, make certain that your youth has the skills and abilities to accomplish the goals.

The most straightforward example is probably that of an ADHD youth. By definition, ADHD youth are disorganized. That is one of the symptoms of the disorder. It is not that ADHD teenagers *won't* get organized, it is that they often *can't* get organized because they don't know where to begin, how to keep things organized, and how to stay focused on the task and not get distracted. In cases such as this, parents need to sit down and plan out with the youth how to organize homework tasks to be done, how to schedule breaks in the work, and how to keep track of what is done and what remains to be finished before setting up a rewards program for getting homework done. With some ADHD teens, the very first reward may not be for getting the homework done; it may simply be for setting up an organized way to accomplish doing the homework.

Borrowing from Barkley and colleagues (1999), there are certain essential principles about both negative and positive consequences. First, positive or negative consequences need to be as immediate as possible. Teenagers live in the moment. Increasingly, this is due to the hurried and pressured life that teenagers lead today. It is also due to the fact that teenagers have not yet matured to an adult status. Having problems with delayed gratification is normal. Only as they age, will youth be better able to delay gratification. To ask a thirteen-year-old to delay gratification is, except in the most rare of circumstances, asking that youth to do that which is nearly impossible for him or her. So, to ask a youth to make the connection between a behavior that occurred days, hours, or even minutes before the consequence is more often than not setting that youth up for failure to recognize and learn from the association between behavior and consequence. Consequences, be they positive or negative, need to be immediate. The more delayed the consequence, the more ineffective it will be.

Consequences need to be focused, reliable, and regular. When a youth does something that either earns a reward or a negative consequence, the consequence needs to be focused only on that behavior. Thus, when a youth is defiant and refuses to go to bed, the consequence should be only for that and the parent needs to resist the temptation to throw in an "Oh, by the way, I remember what you did last week" consequence. It is similar to marriage counseling when arguing couples are told to stick to the subject. The focus should be on the issue at hand and only that issue. Bickering couples should argue only about the immediate subject, not bring up old hurts and prior actions. This is called "gunnysacking," carrying around all of your old hurts and bad feelings in a gunnysack on your back and unloading them whenever you get into a fight with your significant other. The same goes for parents and kids. The reward should be focused on only one targeted behavior. The same is true for punishment. The youth should receive a focused consequence for that one and only transgression, not any others that might have taken place, even just a few minutes earlier.

Reliable consequences mean that both the youth and the parents can count on the fact that what has been promised to happen will happen. When a youth is told that a reward will follow, then it needs to follow. Parents need to follow through on their promises. If they do not, then a mixed and conflicted message is sent to the youth about the importance of keeping one's word. Beyond that, basic research into the use of rewards and punishment demonstrates that if the consequences are not reliable and predictable, then learning will simply not take place, especially at the beginning of the training period. Even more basic than this is the importance of maintaining the reward with the positive behavior and the punishment with the negative behavior.

Often in families that I see due to problems with a youth who is defiant and oppositional, it becomes clear fairly quickly that parents tend to mix up the consequences. They will, for a variety of reasons, forget to reward the positive behaviors in a reliable way. Even more damaging, they may sometimes allow or ignore negative behavior and still give the youth the reward even though the behavior of the youth is exactly the opposite of what is desired. Sometimes this happens because of the press of life. Discipline is not convenient and sometimes parents feel too rushed, they have too little time, or feel that the disruption created by the punishment will be so great that it is simply not worth it in the short run. The problem, of course, is in the long run. When parents are irregular in applying consequences, the youth have little opportunity to make the specific association between the positive behavior and the reward.

Further, it is often the case that in families who have children with anger problems that family life is often chaotic. The source of that chaos is often the angry outbursts of the youth or the fear of the other family members of that outburst. The angry and oppositional youth quickly learns that chaos can bring reward. If the house is kept in a constant state of uproar, he or she is in control. Even if he or she acts in a way totally opposite of how his or her parents want the youth to act, if he or she keeps up the pressure and the confusion, the parents will likely cave in and give the youth what he or she wants. Therefore, even in the face of chaos and time pressures, parents need to actively slow down and maintain control. In reality, there is generally always time for appropriate discipline. Instead, parents make a choice to allow the demands upon their time to determine how they respond to their children. With rare exception, most of those demands are hardly as important as discipline. In the majority of cases, parents can and should take charge of their time and that of their family. In those few cases when that is not possible, it is best to simply do what they can and then deal with it later. But, such events should be the exception, not the rule. Typically, though, in many families, the reverse is true and an essential step for parents is to take control and make certain that both positive and negative consequences are reliable in application.

Regularity in consequences means that positive and negative consequences need to be consistent in order to be effective. Consequences need to be consistent over time, across situations, and by the various people who may give them. Using an example from residential treatment facilities for youth, it is often found in those agencies that have a great deal of problem behaviors, such as aggressive behavior, disobedience to staff, and running away, that there is a great deal of inconsistency in how consequences are given out.

I recall being asked to consult at one residential treatment center for adolescents that seemed to be completely out of control. There were daily physical fights between staff and youth, and youth were sneaking off campus to smoke cigarettes and abuse substances. The first thought of the staff responsible for the program was to say that the kids that had been referred into the program were untreatable. The staff said that the kids came from very delinquent backgrounds, were "treatment failures," or were "developing antisocial personalities and criminals for which there is no treatment." The problem with these arguments was that there was another facility, not that far away, nearly identical in staff and program design, which took virtually the same types of kids from the very same referral sources as the first facility. This made it impossible for the problem to be the kids. They were coming from the same place, had the same experiences, the same types of problems, and the same backgrounds. They were, essentially, identical. Neither was the program the problem. Both agencies had well-thought-out, well-designed counseling and behavioral-management programs. Both had well-trained staff members and a good school. Both had the same staff-to-youth ratio.

Again, on the face of things, both programs were identical. What differed was the application of the program. The agency that didn't have problems made certain that no difference existed between how problems were handled on first, second, and third shifts. All staff members were held strictly accountable to the program in how they were to give out consequences. The administrators held regular reviews to ensure that consequences were consistent across the shifts and that no difference occurred between how third shift and first shift responded to the same type of problem. Moreover, the rewards and consequences followed the youth no matter where they went. The consequences were the same in the school, the residential or living unit, and on any community trips. Finally, and most important, each staff member was closely supervised and routinely evaluated to make certain that the he or she followed the program rules. No inconsistency, no playing of "favorites," and no manipulation of the staff by the kids in the program was tolerated. The staff recognized the importance of consistency and regularity of consequence and believed it to be the most important part of the treatment program.

In clear contrast, the agency with problems was extremely inconsistent in how it applied consequences, both positive and negative. There was a marked difference between the first and second shifts. Kids could get away with all sorts of negative behavior on first shift and in the school. However, the second shift went strictly by the book. When a look was taken at the third shift, it appeared that those staff members had written their own set of rules and disregarded most of the programming of the other two shifts. No wonder the youth's behavior was in chaos, too. The facility itself was in chaos. There was no consistency between the shifts, between the staff members, and in the treatment settings. The youth, lacking any consistent set of program rules and expectations, basically ran the place. The problem, of course, was not with the youth. They were there for treatment and change of exactly this type of behavior. The problem was in the lack of consistency by the staff.

In a way, homes are "residential treatment." Actually, residential treatment centers try to be as homelike as possible. This is not likely a realistic goal since no institution can really be a home. But what is similar is the essential need for regularity and consistency in consequences. Parents need to agree beforehand on the rules and expectations and must agree to follow them to the letter. If there is a disagreement between parents, such disagreements should be worked out either before or after the problem, never in the midst of it and most certainly not in front of the youth. If this is not the case, the teenagers will quickly learn that their parents are not serious about this rule or that and will use that to their advantage (again, much as we adults often do—at work, for example). The problem is not that youth push limits. Teenagers do that as a normal and necessary part of growing up. The problem is that the rules are not regular and consistent and are easily bent and broken.

Another situation that often arises is that no matter how parents try to set up a system of rewards and consequences, there always seems to be a situation that is unanticipated or seemingly unplanned. I suggest, borrowing an analogy from football, that parents spend time in a "chalk talk." Whenever possible, parents should anticipate problems and decide in advance how they will respond. If parents simply wait until something happens and then "punt" it is nearly guaranteed that the results will be unsuccessful. Rather, parents should talk between themselves about how to manage situations that might arise. Then, they should sit down with their teenager and spell out specifically and directly what the behavioral expectations are and what the positive consequences and negative consequences will be in that regard.

Not all of life is expected, however. Parents cannot plan for every consequence. Instead of trying to do that, they should agree in advance about a "crisis-management plan." That is, when an unpredicted situation comes up, the parent who must deal with the situation has some agreed-upon guidelines and rules by which to make decisions. The parent makes the best of the situation and that ends it. If the other parent does have a problem with how the first parent handled the situation, that disagreement is never aired in the presence of the youth. The parents wait until a later and calmer time to discuss how the matter was managed. If need be, a set of rules and expectations for the next time such a situation develops can be drawn up.

CONTRACTS

Beyond the age of twelve or thirteen, depending upon the maturity of the youth, the use of point systems begins to be ineffective. Adolescents don't respond well to them because they generally seem too childish. As a result, a different, more age-appropriate approach is called for with middle to older adolescents. The most useful of these approaches is using behavioral contracts. A typical contract specifies that for a desired behavior, a certain positive result will take place. For example, completion of homework on time throughout the week could earn extra sleeping-in time on Sundays. Contracts work well because they clearly spell out what is desired/required and what will follow. They serve as an excellent teaching instrument because some sort of explicit or implicit contract governs most of our adult lives. They also can be used to shape increased autonomy and demonstration of increased responsibility of the youth.

Some specific caveats to the use of contracts are important. Not all of the youth's life should be governed by contracts. Contracts, as with point systems, work when they are focused upon one or two specific behaviors. So, resist the temptation to develop a sheaf of contracts. After all, the prospect of living in a household so full of contracts that a team of attorneys must be on call is probably not too appealing.

Perhaps the most critical part of contracting is the involvement of the youth in the developing of the contract. A sure way to make certain that the strategy does not work is to write out the contract without the youth and then call them in, give them a pen, and tell them to sign it. Think how you would react to such a situation. Your kids are no different. So, the best way to ensure success is to sit down and talk with your teenagers about desired mutual goals. You have a goal of having the teenager's room not be listed on the board of health's hit list. He or she has a goal of becoming the world-renowned authority on *The Simpsons.* Somewhere in there rests a compromise. By sitting down and working out an agreement, you not only give it a better chance of working but you also teach your teenager about negotiation, compromise, and other skills that lead to greater independence.

It is important that contracts be limited to one and just one behavior/expectation. If there are other expectations, I suggest other specific contracts at first, but no more than three. After that, it gets too complicated for the average adult, much less the teenager. After a period of success in the three contracts, it is certainly possible to sit down together and draft a master contract that covers what the three individual contracts addressed. The contract should focus on one expectation and should spell out only one positive and one negative consequence. It should be time-limited and should also allow for renegotiation. A typical contract can follow a format such as that shown in Box 7.1.

GROUNDING

The most effective reward for teenagers is the awarding of extra privileges. As well, the most effective negative consequence is the denial of some sort of privilege. Typically, the negative consequence used is some sort of grounding. Grounding can mean being made to stay at home for a certain time, not being allowed to use the telephone, computer, video games, or a combination of one or more of these privileges. In the overall scheme of things, grounding is typi-

---

Box 7.1. Sample Contract

On _____(date), _____ (youth) and _____
(parent) agree to the following. _____(youth) agrees to
_____. In return, _____ (parent) agrees to
_____. If the youth does not honor the agreement, the
following negative consequence will take place: _____.
If the parent does not honor the agreement, the following negative consequence
will take place: _____

We have read and agreed to this contract. Any changes must be agreed upon
by both parties in writing and we agree to renegotiate the contract if disputes
arise.

_____ (youth)
_____ (parent)

---

cally the most serious negative consequence that a parent can use. For
that reason, it needs to be used in a specific targeted manner and
should not be overused.

Probably the single most important reason that grounding fails is
that parents tend to fall into a cycle in which the youth is grounded for
a specific period of time, misbehaves, and is grounded for a longer
time. This cycle continues until the youth is grounded for such a long
time that he or she simply sees no end to it and figures, "Why
bother?" The effects of extremely long grounding are not just limited
to the youth being punished. Grounding is inconvenient for the parents and can very much limit their freedom. In a cycle in which the
youth has been grounded for an extreme period, parents often find it
simply impossible to totally enforce the grounding and let up after a
while. The result is that the full "sentence" is not served and the consequence eventually becomes meaningless.

In order for grounding to work, it must be a reasonable period of
time. I suggest that grounding only last in the range of two hours to
two days. Any period longer than that is really not practical. Of
course, in determining how long the youth should be grounded, the
seriousness of the misbehavior should be considered. If need be, one

other negative consequence can be added but this should be a rare exception, not the rule.

Grounding needs to be enforced. A parent would generally not expect to ground a youth, then go on a vacation over the weekend and expect that the kid will obediently sit in his or her room and abstain from using the television and so on. When a youth is grounded, at least one adult (preferably two) must be present to enforce the restriction. This makes grounding generally pretty inconvenient, which is another good reason that it should be seen as the last, not the first resort. Because of this, sometimes grounding may need to be delayed. This of course differs from the structure of a point system but often cannot be helped. Rather than seeing this as a disadvantage, some creative parents have gone so far as to impose a "suspended sentence" and probation. That is, the youth is scheduled to be grounded but if he or she is completes some type of "community service," the grounding can be lifted or avoided entirely.

I also suggest that during the time of grounding, the youth be required to perform some duty or chore that is not particularly beloved but is reasonable (e.g., mopping the kitchen floor). Again, the parents may chose to allow the youth to "work off" some of the grounding time by doing chores, if that seems to be appropriate. When youth are grounded, it is not all that realistic to expect that they will be kept totally from some things, such as listening to the radio or listening to CDs that they bought with money they earned. Rather than fight over it, this is a chance for parents to model reasonableness and compromise. But, in such cases, allowing these may make grounding less effective and if you can't reasonably keep your youth from certain things, then perhaps the use of grounding is not the best approach.

Just as with point systems, there is an age when grounding is no longer effective. The "window" for grounding tends to be between the ages of thirteen and sixteen. After that, the level of developmental maturity of the youth often makes grounding ineffective. At that time, withholding of privileges such as the use of the car, or others that the parents do have direct control over can be far more effective.

INDEPENDENCE

As previously mentioned, handing out a negative consequence to a youth or offering a reward for a behavior without teaching the youth the skills to achieve that behavior simply results in setting up that youth to not be successful. In order to achieve a goal, the youth needs to learn the needed steps to accomplish that goal. For the most part, when we look carefully at the needs and desires of the youth that are behind the negative behaviors, we see that most of what kids want is actually a healthy goal of growing up. This is not to say that substance abuse involvement or being sexually active are desired endpoints of adolescence. But when you think about what these behaviors mean, they become more understandable. The goal of adolescent development is increasing independence and the desired result is a capable, functional adult. Even drug abuse and sexual acting out represent a move to greater independence, albeit in an unhealthy and likely damaging way. Because most healthy families would not support active sexual behavior and substance abuse, such behaviors represent a move outside of family boundaries and rules. In this way, so too does getting a part-time job and earning one's own money and learning the ways of the workplace serve as a step toward independence. One way is healthy; the other is not. It is not so much whether teenagers will develop behaviors that move them toward independence. Rather, it is a question of just what types of behaviors they will develop. Because of this, it is imperative that parents both prepare their children for independence and grant it gradually and in a manner appropriate for the age of the youth. After all, the capacities of a seventeen-year-old are far different from the capacities of a thirteen-year-old, no matter how mature that younger adolescent may appear. A thirteen-year-old simply does not have either the cognitive development or the social maturity to manage independence in the same manner as a seventeen-year-old.

With increasing freedom and independence comes increasing responsibility. Parents should give increased freedom only with demonstrated increased responsibility. It is not appropriate for parents to allow greater freedom and wait for increased responsibility to be seen. The opposite is required. Parents should require specific demonstrations of responsible behavior prior to the earning of increased freedom. A good example is the use of a car, or staying out later at night.

Parents should set out a level of increased expectation such as greater participation in completing household chores, responsible watching of younger siblings, or attainment of a certain grade point average before allowing the use of a car.

Granting privileges needs to be structured and sequential. To use the car example, the parents should break down in very specific terms what is expected before the use of the car. These expectations should be listed in specific steps in a graduated manner. Use of it should not be "carte blanche." Rather, use of the car should be given on a gradual basis and time allowed to use it should be based upon demonstration of responsible use of the car and continued demonstration of responsibility at home. In this manner, increased freedom can accomplish both the goal of allowing the youth to fulfill the normal desires of independence and gradually shape and teach responsible behaviors. If the youth, as will most certainly happen, does not demonstrate the next step of responsibility that was outlined, then he or she should remain on the step just before the failed one. Never should the youth be returned to square one, except in grave or potentially dangerous circumstances. When a youth is returned to or kept at a level, the parent should clearly explain why this is happening and what needs to happen in order to move on. No negotiation should occur. Without question, explaining the "whys and hows" of the situation is an essential component of teaching responsibility and independence. Giving in to manipulation teaches just the opposite.

CHOOSE YOUR BATTLES

With adolescents, as well as with younger children, parents need to think in advance about which issues are open for negotiation right now, which issues could be negotiated in the future, and which issues are never open to negotiation. Basically, parents should pick their battles. Certain issues (e.g., house rules or television shows) can be conceded to the youth. These things, in the larger perspective, don't really matter. But most certainly some issues do matter and should never be areas of negotiation. Parents should not negotiate with their youth about physical violence, respecting parents, drug abuse, sexual activity, smoking, or other matters such as cruelty to animals.

Parents can and must set limits. It is important, of course, to clearly state to youth which rules are simply not negotiable and which negative consequences will follow if they are not followed. Often in my practice I see parents who have either been worn down or have simply given up their power and control as parents. Being a parent is not a popularity contest. There will be clear times when as a responsible parent you must set limits and your youth will naturally become quite upset about it. Parents who wish to produce responsible and independent young adults from their teenagers cannot shy away from setting limits, enforcing these limits, and explaining why the limits exist. Explaining limits is vastly different from apologizing for them or even minimizing the expected ill feelings on the part of the youth as a result. But there are bottom lines and parents are responsible for enforcing them. Parents are authorities, not dictators, and enforcing basic rules, although a necessary component of parenting, is not in and of itself sufficient. To run a household based on dictatorship and punishment is not only ineffective discipline, it is also a sure way to produce youth who have any number of psychological and behavioral problems.

When issues are open to discussion, parents can use these moments for teaching and creativity. One quality of teenagers that sadly seems to drop off in most of us as we age is the ability to see new and novel solutions. Teenagers can often see opportunities or strategies that adults cannot. So, when moving past the "bottom line," nonnegotiable issues to those that either can be or could be negotiated in the future, the opportunity for youth to use their creative problem-solving skills in the family is frequently presented. Allowing youth to be creative in problem solving teaches them essential skills for independence and lets the youth know that authority does not mean immobility. Youth learn that by creative problem solving, they can make beneficial changes, however small, in their lives.

At a much more pragmatic level, again just as with adults, teenagers who have been part of developing rules and consequences will be more invested, take more ownership, and will comply much more readily with rules. One important aspect of this process is determining when the youth is an "equal partner" and when the vote of the parent is final. Again, this is an important lesson of life to be learned. Prior to the problem-solving session parents must set out in advance who has the final say. When parents have an angry, oppositional teenager, the teenager often learns that negative behavior is the most effective way to gain desired ends. By gradually allowing and shaping the teenager's participation in important family decisions, parents can begin to show the youth that positive behavior is more effective in the long run than coercion and manipulation through either actual negative behavior or threats.

TALKING IT THROUGH THE FAMILY

Good communication is essential to any family in order to negotiate and solve problems. Parents sometimes make the assumption that their kids know how to speak their minds. (Sometimes it seems that this is all that they do!) However, teenagers are not as skilled as they seem in expressing themselves and most certainly are not skilled listeners. Child and adolescent "experts" often tell parents that teaching good communication skills is a critical part of their job. The problem is that teenagers tend to learn by observing, not by listening. Rarely would a teenager be interested in sitting down to a lecture by his or her parents on communication skills. Communication is a skill taught by doing. Teenagers learn to communicate with their parents by watching their parents communicate with each other and with them. If parents do not effectively listen to each other, how can a teenager be expected to learn good listening skills? Parents need to set up times for discussion, not always about family issues, but about anything and have those discussions in front of the kids. It is not so much what is talked about but how each adult respects and attends to the concerns of the other that is important. The kids may look bored, and may very well be quickly bored, but they are also learning, much more than they may seem.

I also suggest to families that they make certain that family-life discussions take place not just when problems arise. Parents are also managers and they need to know how life is progressing in both good times and in bad. Regular family meetings are an effective way to accomplish this, but other families have discovered creative ways to communicate through innovations ranging from "idea boxes" to "graffiti" walls. Involving your teenager in a discussion about this is an excellent way to allow him or her to demonstrate problem-solving skills.

Perhaps the biggest challenge facing adults is to learn how to communicate with teenagers. Our previous discussions contained great material, but what if the teen simply refuses to communicate? Then what? I have learned in working with teenagers and their families that there are simply times in which you cannot and never will be able to force a teen to talk. When he or she shuts down and sullenly stares away, parents are most likely to go "ballistic." This, of course, is one of the primary reasons their angry kids act out. Anger is all about power and control. Not all anger is expressed directly. Sometimes, the most effective way that an angry teen can use anger is by shutting down and sullenly refusing to talk. No matter how the parent threatens, yells, confronts, or even dances about in a chicken suit, the youth simply refuses to talk.

This is the classic example of a power struggle between an angry, oppositional youth and an adult. Adults forget that they ultimately still hold the power and consequently lose the struggle. True, you cannot make the kid talk, but you can take other actions. The first step is to walk away from the fight. The less you resist, the stronger you become. Simply tell the youth what you think and feel, and state that until he or she chooses to talk about it, there will be no (fill in the blank) privilege. Then, leave it at that. Time is on your side. Or, to use the words of my grandmother once again, "Just because he threw out the bait doesn't mean you have to rise to it." When a child insults or disrespects you, respond nonemotionally; state the issue. The more your youth yells at you, the more you need to keep a calm, level voice as you tell the youth what will happen (or what will not) if he or she doesn't stop yelling. If you need to, take a break, take a walk, and cool down. Do what you need to do to stay composed and in control.

IT'S NOT WHAT IS *THAT MATTERS—*
IT'S WHAT WE BELIEVE

More often than not, what we think about a situation drives how we feel about it. Different people look at the same situation in highly different manners and how they look at a situation often determines how they respond to that situation. I think that we hold a number of beliefs about kids that really are unreasonable and get us into trouble. The first of these is destiny. Far too often, parents look at the current difficult, even obnoxious behavior of their teens and from that standpoint make the dire prediction that their children will be pure failures in the future. If you think about it, most kids never do all of their homework. Most kids do come to class unprepared. Most kids won't get all As. Be glad when something even close to that happens and give praise and rewards bountifully. If you expect your teen to always do homework, you are setting both you and your teen up for a miserable, argument-filled school year. What is actually reasonable to expect? Just how diligent were you, really, in doing your homework? How important is it for your teen to experience the natural and logical consequences of not doing homework (flunking, summer school, detentions). The same goes for family gatherings. Didn't you need your "space" when you were growing up? With few exceptions, would you rather have spent time with your best friend or with your second cousin once removed? How about moodiness? Were you always the picture of happiness as a teen? The same goes for keeping up a room. Although minimum health standards are necessary, can you cite specific research between the relationship of a dirty room and success or lack thereof in later adulthood?

Without fail, I think that we all tend to get caught up in cognitive traps of thinking the worst when the worst is not really what will happen. As an exercise, take a moment and jot down your "catastrophic thoughts" about your teen and decide just how real those worries are.

PROBLEM SOLVING

What if your youth doesn't have a good idea about how to solve problems? We can't just assume that they have somehow, perhaps through osmosis, come up with effective problem-solving strategies. Youth who have ADHD, are oppositional defiant, or who have anger problems typically have considerable trouble problem solving. Often, youth who are chronically angry don't need to develop problem-solving skills. They can get what they want by just acting out or somehow threatening to act out. They don't need to learn problem solving because their use of anger and coercion works just often enough that they don't need to learn any other way. Take away the angry outbursts, and you have a youth who is very limited in ability to solve problems and meet personal needs.

There are many methods of problem solving. One that can be used and modified is shown in Box 7.2. I strongly suggest that parents decide not to hold a lecture. Rather, learn these steps and model them. Think out loud, literally, when you have the chance to model problem-solving behavior.

Regardless of method, teaching effective problem solving can be a useful tool for helping angry and oppositional teens find more productive and useful ways of dealing with situations. Teaching effective problem solving not only helps manage the family life but also equips your teenager with essential skills required for increased independence and responsibility. The importance of problem-solving skills cannot be underestimated.

Box 7.2. Problem-Solving Steps

1. *Be aware of your feelings*—When you attempt to solve a conflict or problem between people, make certain that you are aware of how you feel about the issue and how the other person or persons feel. Ask questions; don't assume. Make certain that each person involved has the chance to clearly speak, without interruption, about how he or she feels about the problem.
2. *Identify the specific problem*—What you might think is the problem may be very different from how the others think. Make certain that each person is clear on the specific problem and that there is a mutual understanding in very basic terms of what the problem is.
3. *Set a clear goal*—Before you try to define solutions, think of where you want to go. Ask the question, "If things were the way we wanted them to be, what would it be like? How would we know?" Allow each person to express his or her version of the best possible situation or outcome. Don't cut off or limit anyone by saying something is not possible.
4. *Think of alternative solutions*—At first, just brainstorm; let any possible solution be listened to and considered. Only after each person feels that he or she has come up with all possible solu-

(continued)

(continued)

tions should you then begin the process of narrowing down these solutions.

5. *Evaluate possible consequences*—Anticipate the results of each of the different choices. Ask, "What would happen if we did . . .?"
6. *Select the best choice*—After listening to each person and drawing out potential consequences, decide which of the alternatives has the most realistic chance of success. If needed, list them in order.
7. *Develop an action plan*—Decide what you need to do and lay out clear and specific steps along the way. Set "benchmarks" or ways to know how you are doing. Anticipate potential roadblocks and devise a plan to deal with them. Look at changes that could or should be made and also try to think of what could go wrong and what to do about it.
8. *Feedback*—Set some times to talk about what is happening or did not happen. Set up feedback times at least midway through the change process and afterward. Feedback should be nonjudgmental observations of what is happening and opinions. Criticism is only useful if constructive and framed in a way that suggests positive change. Feedback that is negative without constructive suggestions or is an attack upon someone is not helpful and should not be allowed. Try to notice any unplanned results from your actions and also see what you have learned along the way.
9. *Learn*—No one method works every time. If the problem isn't solved, step back for a short time and think about how you approached the problem-solving process. Consider if you could have done anything differently and try that next time.

Chapter 8

Building on the Positive

For most of this book, I have focused on the problems that children can present us. That is, regretfully, a common human trait. I imagine most of the readers who have purchased this book have done so because they either have a child with anger-management problems or seek to use this as a resource in their own work with children and families who have problems with anger. We look for solutions to problems when we have them. When we have problems, we become focused on just the problems, often ignoring all the good that can be found in the child or the situation. Thus, we focus on the weaknesses and not the strengths of the child.

We really can't, however, solve a problem by focusing on negative behavior. To do so results in an isolated and often very narrow view of the situation, which limits the possible solutions. I am convinced that focusing and building on the strengths of the person rather than correcting perceived weaknesses or faults solves problems. There are many good reasons for the validity of this approach that extend far beyond simple "feel good" reasons. The validity rests in sound scientific research about therapy outcomes that spans more than two decades.

Beyond all else, what we can count on to improve the quality of their lives and ours is the strength of our youth. Most kids are very resilient. They are able to get through most trials and travails of adolescence with very little scarring. Kids are stronger and more resilient than we typically give them credit for. Parents can do a number of things to enhance that strength, and increase the resilient characteristics of their youth.

STRENGTH BUILDING
AND POSITIVE ROLE MODELS

Parents can promote and encourage healthy attachments and bring into their children's lives persons who will take a positive interest in them. They can expose them to healthy relationships and talk with them about what makes good relationships work. Parents can encourage pet ownership and pet responsibility as a stepping-stone to lasting relationships with others. Many times in my practice with children who have suffered considerable emotional and/or physical abuse, it is not I but my dog, C. J., who makes the first meaningful therapeutic contact with a well-planned and totally irresistible wag of his tail. Parents can do whatever they need to do to make certain that their relationships are healthy ones.

Most of all, as I have stressed throughout this book, kids learn by observing: they learn not by what we say, but by what we do. For that reason, exposure to positive role models is vital. Role models can come from their own relationships or from the media. Wherever they come from, these role models are vital in shaping the young person's perceptions and expectations of the world. For that reason, parents must limit what children see on television, movies, and in video games. They must take charge of the terrible and proven effect of violence in the media, limiting the media exposure of their children both at home and with peers. Of course, children can never be completely sheltered from these influences, but parents can teach them the difference between fantasy and reality. Rather than simply saying that such violent role models are "bad" and should be avoided, parents should explain why they are to be shunned. Parents should point out the difference between what it is really like to be a victim of violence and how it is portrayed in the mass media. In this regard, kids should be rewarded for making positive choices about what they watch and which games they play. Rather than focusing on what is forbidden, parents should notice and appreciate when their kids actually chose appropriate shows, songs, and video games.

DIVERSITY AND THE POWER OF OTHERS

Other well-recognized causes of violence are hate, misunderstanding, and prejudice. Children are not born hating others. They are not born with inherent prejudice. These beliefs and actions are learned from adults. Diversity comes not just from exposure to other cultures and individuals. It comes from building understanding and appreciation of differences. The lack of prejudice flows from the development of understanding and empathy for other cultures. In building this sort of bridge, differences become not frightening and threatening but welcoming and exciting to children. Children can be exposed to and encouraged to learn about others at an early age. This can start at a family level with extended family members and evolve into learning about others in the neighborhood, school, churches, and the larger community. Children can explore other cultures not only through direct experience but also by using the positive power of the media through books, television, movies, and video games. (Yes, there are a number of nonviolent, socially positive games. They just don't get the press.)

Another way to ensure that your child grows to appreciate others is to not only expose him or her to different cultures and lifestyles, but to teach your child to listen. It is hard enough to learn to listen to those similar to us. Listening to others who are unlike us takes even more skill and concentration. A person can, after all, listen but not "hear." In cross-cultural situations, ask what he or she learned. Teach the concept of listening with understanding, not with assumptions. Listening is a skill, one that we must always work on. By exposing your child to listening with understanding to different cultures and their heritages, you too are practicing and developing your skills. Share that experience with your child.

VALUES

Do not be afraid of your values or of teaching them to your children. Children need to learn core values and, as always, they learn by observing and watching. In the time that you spend with your children, talk about moral choices you make on a daily basis. When you watch television, talk about the moral choices portrayed. Remember when you do this that young children look at the world in very concrete either/or terms. Only gradually can they move to the more abstract and philosophical views that we as adults have. There is nothing bad about a firm foundation of right and wrong. Whatever your code or core values are, they should be taught to your children. No one expects children to completely accept those values. At some point they will, of course, rebel against them. Curiously, in the case of many youth, the stronger the rebellion, the more completely they embrace those values as they mature.

Parents need to consistently look for ways to teach children non-violent problem-solving strategies and notice and reward them when kids actually put those strategies into place. At first, the sources of power over a child are the parents, the extended family, the neighborhood, and then school. As the child matures, that source moves inward and he or she evolves into an independent, self-motivated person.

We all want to continue to expose our children to nonviolent, morally correct experiences and shield them from the opposite. But, as we well know, this is not always feasible or possible. In such cases, we can teach our children where to look even within the most negative situations. To illustrate at a very basic level, although crime is higher in the poorest parts of our cities, not all of the people who live there are criminals. Deep within our strife-torn urban centers are decent, honorable, and honest people. Frankly, there are more of them than the criminals. Children who live within those settings face terrible negative influences that they often cannot avoid. They not only need to learn hope, self-motivation, and control, but also how to seek out and associate with the healthy persons and segments of their community. For some, this skill is the difference between life and death.

For those of us who are blessed with not having our children face such terrible choices, we must realize that on a less dramatic but no less important scale, our children make the same kinds of choices. Every day at school, your child chooses a peer group, choosing to associate or not associate with certain peers. This is not an inherent ability. It is a learned skill that we teach our children and should also notice, appreciate, and reward when we see it taking place.

Children should learn certain strategies to avoid habitually responding in angry, potentially violent ways. They should learn to keep an open mind about differences in others, and take time to learn and listen. It is important that we teach our children how to laugh and have a sense of humor. As previously discussed, parents can make mental catastrophes out of events that really are not all that important. They think the worst, expect the worst, and are not surprised when that self-fulfilling prophecy comes to full realization. For that reason, teaching kids to take a moment to step back and question their assumptions can lead to looking at the world without anger as the first emotional response.

Parents can teach children to slow down and look at new situations with a first response of peacefulness and nonaggression. In doing this, they are not teaching children to deny or minimize the true dangers of our society. Rather, parents are teaching children to choose what cues to respond to and how. By teaching them to slow down, reflect, and think of alternatives, potential cues to anger and violence can be reduced, surroundings can be controlled, and the world can be seen in a humanizing rather than a depersonalizing manner. After all, what is the world is ours; what the world will be rests in the promise of our children.

Bibliography

American Academy of Child and Adolescent Psychiatry (1999). *Fact sheet on attention deficit hyperactivity disorder.* Washington, DC: American Academy of Child and Adolescent Psychiatry.

American Psychiatric Association (1994). *Diagnostic and statistical manual of mental disorders,* Fourth edition. Washington, DC: American Psychiatric Association.

American Psychiatric Association (2000). *Diagnostic and statistical manual of mental disorders,* Fourth edition, Text revision. Washington, DC: American Psychiatric Association.

American Psychological Association (1993). *Violence and youth: Psychology's response.* Washington, DC: American Psychological Association.

American Psychological Association (2001). *Adults and children together against violence.* Washington, DC: American Psychological Association.

American Psychological Association (2002). *ACT training program: Program implementation handbook.* Washington, DC: The American Psychological Association.

Austin, J., Johnson, K., and Gregoria, M. (2000). *Juveniles in adult prisons and jails: A national assessment.* Washington, DC: United States Department of Justice, Bureau of Justice Assistance.

Bandura, A. and Shunk, D.H. (1981). Cultivating competence, self-efficacy, and intrinsic interest through proximal self-motivation. *Journal of Personality and Social Psychology,* 41: 586-598.

Barkley, R.A. (1995). *Taking charge of ADHD.* New York: The Guilford Press.

Barkley, R.A. (1997). *Defiant children: A clinician's manual for assessment and parent training,* Second edition. New York: The Guilford Press.

Barkley, R.A. (1998). *ADHD: A handbook for diagnosis and treatment,* Second edition. New York: The Guilford Press.

Barkley, R.A., Edwards, G.H., and Robin, A.L. (1999). *Defiant teens: A clinician's manual for assessment and family intervention.* New York: The Guilford Press.

Beck, A. and Harrison, P. (2000). *Prisoners in 2000.* Washington, DC: United States Department of Justice, Bureau of Justice Statistics.

Bender, L. (1959). Children and adolescents who kill. *American Journal of Psychiatry,* 116: 410-413.

Benedek, E.P. (1992). Adolescent homicide: Victims and victimizers. In Schetky, D.H. and Benedek, E.P. (Eds.), *Clinical handbook of child psychiatry and law* (pp. 216-229). Baltimore, MD: Williams and Wilkins.

Bowlby, J. (1971). *Attachment and loss,* Volume 1: *Attachment.* New York: Pelican.

Bridges, K.M.B. (1933). A study of social development in early infancy. *Child Development,* 4: 36-39.

Calicchia, J., Moncata, S., and Santostefano, S. (1993). Cognitive control differences in violent juvenile inpatients. *Journal of Clinical Psychology,* 49(5): 731-740.

Erikson, E.H. (1959). *Identity and the life cycle: Selected papers.* New York: International Universities Press.

Green, R.W. (1998). *The explosive child.* New York: HarperCollins.

Kohlberg, L. (1976). Moral stages and moralization: The cognitive-developmental approach. In Lickona, T. (Ed.), *Moral development and behavior* (pp. 83-120). New York: Holt, Rinehart, and Winston.

National Institute of Mental Health (1996). *Attention deficit hyperactivity disorder* Washington, DC: United States Government Printing Office.

Olweus, D. (1993). *Bullying at school: What we know and what we can do.* Malden, MA: Blackwell.

Patterson, G.R., Capaldi, D., and Bank, L. (1991). An early starter model for predicting delinquency. In Pepler, D.J. and Ruben, K.H. (Eds.), *The development and treatment of childhood aggression* (pp. 139-168). Hillsdale, NJ: Lawrence Erlbaum Associates.

Patterson, G.R., DeBaryshe, B.D., and Ransey, E. (1989). A developmental perspective on antisocial behavior. *The American Psychologist,* 44(2): 329-335.

Pepler, D.J. and Slaby, R.G. (1994). Theoretical and developmental perspectives on youth and violence. In Eron, L.D., Gentry, J.H., and Schlegel, P. (Eds.), *Reason to hope: A psychosocial perspective on violence and youth* (pp. 27-58). Washington, DC: American Psychological Association.

Phenlan, T. (1996). *1,2,3 magic: Effective discipline for children ages 2-12.* Glen Elyn, IL: Child Management, Inc.

Piaget, J. (1963). *The origins of intelligence in children.* New York: Norton.

Quinn, M.M., Jannasch-Pennell, A., and Rutherford, R.B. (1995). Using peers as social skills training agents for students with antisocial behavior: A cooperative learning approach. *Preventing School Failure,* 39: 26-31.

Reid, J.B. and Patterson, G.R. (1989). The development of antisocial behavior patterns in childhood and adolescence. *European Journal of Psychology,* 2(19): 107-119.

Satcher D. (1999a). *Mental health: A report of the surgeon general.* Washington DC: United States Department of Health and Human Services, Office of the Surgeon General.

Satcher D. (1999b). *Youth violence: A report of the surgeon general.* Washington DC: United States Department of Health and Human Services, Office of the Surgeon General.

Snyder, H. and Sickmund, M. (1999). *Juvenile offenders and victims: 1999 national report.* Washington DC: Office of Juvenile Justice and Delinquency Prevention.

Spitz, R.A. (1945). Hospitalism: An inquiry into the genesis of psychiatric conditions in early childhood. In A. Freud et al. (Eds.), *Psychoanalytic study of the child* (pp. 53-74). New York: International Universities Press.

Turecki, S. and Tonner, L. (2000). *The difficult child.* New York: Bantam Books.

Villani, S. (2001). Impact of media on children and adolescents: A 10-year review of the research. *Journal of the American Academy of Child and Adolescent Psychiatry,* 40: 4.

Index

SPECIAL 25%-OFF DISCOUNT!
Order a copy of this book with this form or online at:
http://www.haworthpress.com/store/product.asp?sku=5006

YOUR ANGRY CHILD
A Guide for Parents

_____in hardbound at $22.46 (regularly $29.95) (ISBN: 0-7890-1223-5)

_____in softbound at $11.21 (regularly $14.95) (ISBN: 0-7890-1224-3)

Or order online and use special offer code HEC25 in the shopping cart.

COST OF BOOKS_____

OUTSIDE US/CANADA/
MEXICO: ADD 20%_____

POSTAGE & HANDLING_____
(US: $5.00 for first book & $2.00
for each additional book)
(Outside US: $6.00 for first book
& $2.00 for each additional book)

SUBTOTAL_____

IN CANADA: ADD 7% GST_____

STATE TAX_____
(NY, OH, MN, CA, IN, & SD residents,
add appropriate local sales tax)

FINAL TOTAL_____
(If paying in Canadian funds,
convert using the current
exchange rate, UNESCO
coupons welcome)

☐ **BILL ME LATER:** ($5 service charge will be added)
(Bill-me option is good on US/Canada/Mexico orders only;
not good to jobbers, wholesalers, or subscription agencies.)

☐ Check here if billing address is different from
shipping address and attach purchase order and
billing address information.

Signature_____

☐ **PAYMENT ENCLOSED: $**_____

☐ **PLEASE CHARGE TO MY CREDIT CARD.**

☐ Visa ☐ MasterCard ☐ AmEx ☐ Discover
☐ Diner's Club ☐ Eurocard ☐ JCB

Account # _____

Exp. Date_____

Signature_____

Prices in US dollars and subject to change without notice.

NAME_____

INSTITUTION_____

ADDRESS_____

CITY_____

STATE/ZIP_____

COUNTRY_____ COUNTY (NY residents only)_____

TEL_____ FAX_____

E-MAIL_____

May we use your e-mail address for confirmations and other types of information? ☐ Yes ☐ No
We appreciate receiving your e-mail address and fax number. Haworth would like to e-mail or fax special
discount offers to you, as a preferred customer. **We will never share, rent, or exchange your e-mail address
or fax number.** We regard such actions as an invasion of your privacy.

Order From Your Local Bookstore or Directly From
The Haworth Press, Inc.
10 Alice Street, Binghamton, New York 13904-1580 • USA
TELEPHONE: 1-800-HAWORTH (1-800-429-6784) / Outside US/Canada: (607) 722-5857
FAX: 1-800-895-0582 / Outside US/Canada: (607) 771-0012
E-mailto: orders@haworthpress.com
PLEASE PHOTOCOPY THIS FORM FOR YOUR PERSONAL USE.
http://www.HaworthPress.com   BOF03